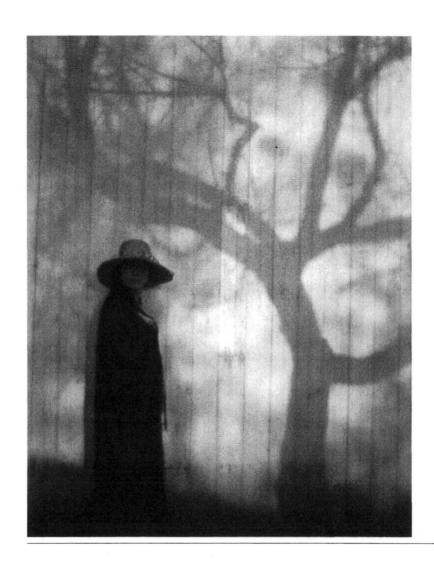

Season
ESSAYS / BRENDA MILLER of the
Body

Sarabande Books

LOUISVILLE, KENTUCKY

No part of this book may be reproduced without written permission of the
publisher. Please direct inquiries to:

> Managing Editor
> Sarabande Books, Inc.
> 2234 Dundee Road, Suite 200
> Louisville, KY 40205

LIBRARY OF CONGRESS CATALOGING-IN-PUBLICATION DATA

Miller, Brenda Lynn, 1959–
    Season of the body : essays / by Brenda Miller.
    p.   cm.
    ISBN 1-889330-68-X (cloth : alk. paper) — ISBN 1-889330-69-8 (pbk. : alk. paper)
1. Miller, Brenda Lynn, 1959– 2. Miller, Brenda Lynn, 1959—-Journeys. 3. Masseurs—United
States—Biography. 4. Jews—United States—Biography. I. Title.
CT275.M51435 A3 2002
615.8'22'092—dc21
[B]   2001040021

Cover image: *Prologue to a Sad Spring, 1920* by Edward Weston © 1981 Center for
Creative Photography, Arizona Board of Regents (see frontispiece for photograph
reproduced in its entirety)

Cover and text design by Charles Casey Martin

Manufactured in the United States of America
This book is printed on acid-free paper.

Sarabande Books is a nonprofit literary organization.

Funded in part by a grant from the Kentucky Arts Council, a state agency of the
Education, Arts, and Humanities Cabinet

FIRST EDITION
Third Printing

For Sean, Hannah, and Sarah

Table of Contents

PART THREE

Acknowledgments

The author gratefully acknowledges the publications where these essays first appeared:

The Georgia Review: "A Thousand Buddhas"
Prairie Schooner: "Basha Leah"
Willow Springs: "Needlepoint"
The Sun: "The Date" and "Infant Ward"
Northern Lights: "Gourd" and "Grape Hyacinths"
Seneca Review: "A Brief History of Sex"
The Bellingham Review: "Season of the Body"
In Brief: Short Takes on the Personal (W.W. Norton, 1999):
    "Artifacts"
Fourth Genre: Explorations in Nonfiction: "How to Meditate"
The Journal: "The Names" (Winner of the William Allen Prize
    in Creative Nonfiction)
Seattle Weekly: "Prologue to a Sad Spring"
Weber Studies: "Next Year in Jerusalem"
Shenandoah: "A Field Guide to the Desert"
Witness: "Time With Children"
Brevity: "Split"

"A Thousand Buddhas" appears in *The Pushcart Prize Anthology XIX: The Best of the Small Presses, 1994/95; Storming Heaven's Gate: An Anthology of Spiritual Writings by Women* (Penguin, 1997); *The Pushcart Book of Essays;* and a special fifty-year anniversary issue of

The Georgia Review anthologizing the best essays that have appeared in its pages over the years. "The Date" is reprinted in *The Beacon Best of 1999: Creative Writing by Women and Men of All Colors* (Beacon Press, 1999). "Basha Leah" appears in *The Pushcart Prize Anthology XXIV: The Best of the Small Presses*, 2000.

Quotations in the essay "Basha Leah" are taken from *The Dictionary of Jewish Lore and Legend* by Alan Unterman (Thames & Hudson, 1991).

The author would like to thank the following foundations and residencies for valuable time and resources for writing this book: The Ludwig Vogelstein Foundation, The Steffenson-Cannon Foundation, The Abraham Woursell Foundation, The Ucross Foundation, The Corporation of Yaddo, Hedgebrook Foundation, and The Millay Colony for the Arts. I am most grateful, as well, for the support and guidance of numerous friends along the way, especially Karen Brennan, Jacqueline Osherow, Connie Voisine, Joel Long, Robert Van Wagoner, John D'Agata, Suzanne Paola, Bruce Beasley, Kristin Bloomer, Keith Scribner, Kathleen Halme, and Ruth Kennedy. Thanks, also, to the team at Sarabande, whose editorial guidance has been a blessing.

I am too alone in the world, and not alone enough
to make every minute holy. . . .
I want to describe myself
like a painting that I looked at
closely for a long time,
like a saying that I finally understood,
like the pitcher I use every day,
like the face of my mother,
like a ship
that took me safely
through the wildest storm of all.

—Rainer Maria Rilke
trans. by Robert Bly

Season of the Body

PROLOGUE

Body Language

FOR A BRIEF TIME, WHEN I WAS IN COLLEGE at Berkeley, *Body Language* was all the rage. My roommates and I passed around a dog-eared copy of the popular book by Julius Fast, thumbing through it with a fervor decidedly lacking in the rest of our studies. It was the seventies, after all, an era of fierce self-scrutiny, and *Body Language* seemed an opportune phrase book for this hazardous terrain. We sat sprawled on the tweedy chairs in the parlor and set about analyzing every tilt of the head, each wave of the hand, various wiggles of the foot. Arms crossed over the chest? Closed-minded, defensive, resistant. The biting of a thumbnail? Obvious regression to infant fear. We caught ourselves twirling stray bits of hair and froze, knowing we'd just given away either boredom or sexual excitement, depending on the angle our knees had assumed.

Though it all seems rather pedestrian now, we gleefully lit into this language like children with secret decoder rings. For weeks, we gazed at each other with frank assessment, taking in all the cues

3

that now, once revealed, would clarify all our efforts at communication. And communication, for us earnest, young college students, meant everything—*everything!* We craved truth in all its various forms, and while we knew we could dissemble easily enough with language, the body always gives us away. Perhaps that's why we latched on to this fleshy lexicon in the first place, knowing our spoken words served as paltry vehicles for all the truths we longed to express. We stayed up late in the night, burning candles and incense, and watched our bodies offer hints from our pasts or clues to our murky futures. We watched ourselves in the mirror of the coed bathroom, wiping away the mist, to divine our deepest, most covert, desires.

This could last only so long. In fact, once unleashed, our bodies jabbered so loudly the din became unbearable. It was only a matter of time before we started to avoid the living room; we threw on bulky army jackets and slunk out the door before catching anyone's eye. We now wanted, with sinking hearts, to muffle these bodies that insisted, like toddlers, on babbling our shame and our secrets. One of us sold the tattered book to Moe's, and we began to ignore our bodies except for the pleasures they might provide, relegating them back to a disgruntled silence, where they belonged.

Several years later—post-college and still searching for an apt livelihood—I enrolled in massage school and learned a new type of body language. Every morning I drove dirt roads from my house in the country to a drafty, two-room building on the outskirts of Willits. A single rosebush waved outside the window, blooming that entire fall. Nine others joined me there—young, hardy people with names like Wolfgang and Starr and Michaela. Eventually I would see these people in the most compromising positions: curled naked on the massage table, sobbing, or crouched on the carpet, their hands clutching at their hair. But that first day they all looked briskly competent; their hands, when they shook my own, felt strong, tender, and forgiving.

Our teacher, Dami, carried a six-month-old girl swaddled to her back. She herded us all into a circle and asked us to close our eyes, breathe deeply, and begin to be aware of the inner lining of our bodies, of each sensation from the top of our heads to the bottoms of our feet. She explained how the muscles cache all the emotions a person suppresses in her life: anger, for instance, lodges in the big muscles of the arms and legs; sorrow lives deep in the chest; doubt drags down the shoulders and bends the spine. A good massage therapist, she said, must first learn to read the body the way one learns to read music, a language of esoteric notation decipherable only to those with talent and proper training.

We opened our eyes and glanced sidelong at each other, already—in the first hour!—chagrined and embarrassed at all our bodies revealed. Dami chose me as an example. She circled silently, her eyes grimly focused on my abdomen, then laid one hand low on my belly. "Look," she said to the class, who leaned forward and looked closely. "See here, how her back sways, her stomach distends. It's as if she's a child, frozen in the posture of a child." She placed her other hand on the dip of my lower back, so that for a moment I was sandwiched between her large palms. "Your job," she told the class, "would be to help this woman release whatever's retarding her emotional life."

My face burned while the class nodded in sage agreement, eyeing my body with renewed interest. When Dami turned to another student, I tried to suck in my stomach, which suddenly looked, to me, inflated as a balloon. I felt the ache in my lower back—a dull pain, I realized then, had needled me for years. My abdomen still tingled from the touch of Dami's hand; she had placed her palm, with deadly accuracy, over the scar left from two miscarriages I'd suffered when I was twenty years old. These pregnancies had torn me apart, bodily and emotionally, but after a few months and a little counseling I'd convinced myself I'd gotten over it. Now, while the rest of the class gazed somberly at Wolfgang's concave chest, I placed one hand on my belly and kept it there, regarding my body with a strange mix of curiosity, anger, and dismay.

In the following weeks, I studied hard. I opened my *Anatomy Coloring Book* and got out my crayons. I learned the musculature of the human body, starting with the easy muscles of the back. I filled in with lilac the voluptuous stretch of latissimus dorsi. I murmured *cervical, thoracic, lumbar,* and *sacrum,* all the while scribbling away with my crayons: intercostals green, pectorals pink. All of this seemed vaguely familiar: I remembered how, as a child, I spent hours with the *Encyclopedia Britannica,* lifting and settling the translucent strata of the body, watching it swell from bare bone to a multilayered organism of blood, nerves and skin. Now I memorized reflexology charts, equating the ball of the foot with the sinuses, the arch with the spine, the heel to the buttocks. I looked at my own bare feet and saw the pituitary in the center of the big toe, the ovaries suspended from the anklebone.

We quickly grew fluent in this new language, learning how to read the bodies before us, to divine at a glance the emotions betrayed by the clenched jaw or the clamp of a quadriceps. We stood quietly by the table, our partner's back exposed, the knobs of vertebrae forming a bright arrow to the center of the body. We cupped one hand on the sacrum ("holy bone" in Greek), and stood there waiting for the body's pulse to beat against our palms. We learned many different kinds of strokes—effleurage, percussion, acupressure, Trager—and we practiced these moves on each other. We rocked the belly, we pressed the sacral ridge, we tapped the clavicle, all the while trying to listen, just listen, to what the body might want to reveal.

Sometimes one person began to cry—husky sobs that triggered respondent cries from massage tables around the room. We rarely spoke to one another during these sessions, except for a whispered reminder to breathe, but the room grew full of so much clamor, we had to flee outdoors afterward and run our hands through cold water. Sometimes I found my compatriots weeping in the bathroom, or on the bench near the perpetually blooming rosebush. My own crying I often did in the car on the way to and from the classroom, gazing blearily at the passing scenery, lost in a grief I thought I had long surmounted.

After I graduated from Dami's classroom, I gave hundreds of massages to clients at a hot springs resort near Mendocino. I used a massage room on the banks of the Big River. Gallon jugs of almond oil crowded the cabinet, and sometimes a vase of cut roses appeared on the windowsill. I massaged many different bodies, each with its own difficult history, its puzzle of a heart. Each time I began by touching the sacrum, that holy bone; when I did so, I often felt myself in the realm of the sacred, tapping into a current of muted benediction.

I remember one time a woman disrobed to reveal a missing breast, the left side of her chest smooth and glossy with scars. We did not speak at all about it, and when she lay down I moved my hand carefully up her calves, then her thighs. I did not ask questions, only whispered the word *breathe* as I headed into the arch of her foot, or the declination of her cheekbones. I touched her chest only at the very end of the massage; I cupped my palms on her sternum, and felt the absence there, an ache traveling up my arm and into my own breast. We both started to cry then: not in a debilitating way, but gently, almost happily, as if we spoke a language of the female, body-to-body, unhampered by the tired obstacle of speech.

It was exhausting work. After a full day of massage, my body sometimes seemed permeable and translucent as silk. I gave up after six years and became a writer instead—a work no less tiring, really, and requiring the same inclination to listen with a hand pressed to the holy bone, to hear the thrum of the body and all it longs to tell. As I wrote, I found myself mapping a history of myself as a history of my body: my female body, with all its scars and beauty marks, its imperfect love beating away inside the chest.

On my writing desk I've propped a photograph called *The West Wind*, shot by Anne Brigman in 1915. From behind, we see a naked woman running headlong across a stormy beach. She stretches a fluttering white veil above her head while her feet skip into the foam of the incoming tide. Her back arcs against the black cliffs and the roiling clouds in the distance. The woman's face, hidden from us, might be somber or afraid, but we'd find a frown unnatural on such a body, one so willing to go down to the water's edge. More than willing, she rushes toward whatever sand and spray might assail her there, welcoming the world and all the traces it leaves behind.

The body knows a language the mind never wholly masters. This woman is naked and alive, in motion on the brink of the known world. Danger surely lurks in such a venture, but the expression of her body spells out happiness of the greatest kind.

PART ONE

Needlepoint

I.

WHEN I WAS TWENTY YEARS OLD, and recovering from emergency surgery, my mother gave me a needlepoint kit. The design was New England in the fall: manicured fields, a farmhouse, russet hills that grew warm under the work of my hands. An embryo had lodged in my fallopian tube and grown, without my being aware of it; one morning it simply ruptured through the narrow duct. I woke in my mother's car as it sped toward the emergency room, my face turned against the gray Naugahyde of the backseat. The pain in my abdomen spread into my chest, my hands, my throat.

I remember the surgical nurse as she appeared above me, her head blocking out the white light of the operating dome. "Do you know this operation could make you sterile?" she asked, her voice muffled through her mask. Already I was counting back from one hundred, the anesthesia coaxing me to sleep, but even through my fog I understood the nurse's question as political more than personal—the year was 1979, and this nurse saw a young woman strapped down on a gurney in a roomful of men with knives. She saw a woman powerless and flat on her back, invisible except for her shaved pubic mound exposed between the sheets. I don't know what she wanted me to say at that moment, or what she expected to do if I shook my head no. The nurse disappeared as my gurney was turned away. As it turned out, another ectopic pregnancy, just nine months later, would make of this nurse a prophet; in later years I would mull on that word, *sterile*, and envision myself as a piece of gleaming steel, pure and invulnerable.

But, as I recovered from surgery, I thought only of that needle-point, each stitch, one after the other, and mounds of color gradually developed under my hands. The simple pattern required only the simplest of stitches—in and out, up and down, slanting first one way, and then the other. The yarn moved through my fingers; the canvas softened as I filled in thousands of tiny squares. I lay in my childhood bed, propped up with pillows against the headboard. I kept the TV on, a small black-and-white RCA tuned to *All My Children* and *Jeopardy!* and *The Mary Tyler Moore Show*. Occasionally I would laugh, but not often because laughing pulled the stitches on the incision across my pelvis. Sometimes I would cry, but that hurt too, so eventually all I did was stitch that needlepoint—in and out, up and down.

Sometimes I became so focused on detail—on one small square of orange, and the square next to it, half orange, half brown, and the one next to that all green—that I was surprised, when I looked up and refocused my gaze, to see I had actually created anything—a blazing hillside of red sugar maples, or a calm stream covered with golden leaves, or the bright white steeple of a church.

II.

Sixteen years later, I've come to Vermont to watch the leaves as they turn. Every night the ground freezes, and by day the sky thickens; at times the sun appears and lights up a single red tree, or cuts a swath through a clump of golden maples. The cold burns my cheeks, and I keep my hands buried deep in my pockets as I walk. I can smell wood burning, and the ripening of apples. I walk carefully, slowly, as if following complicated instructions.

I've just left a man I've lived with for the last five years. The pain of this separation is difficult to identify—it's physical, but not rooted in the body; it flits about my chest and wobbles through my abdomen. I try to describe it to my friend Kristin. Kristin is taller than I am; she has strong arms, short blond hair, and a gaze that locks onto mine. She holds my hand as we walk. I tell her about the years Keith and I spent together, about the trivial things I took for proof of permanence—the coffee brought to bed in the mornings, the bicycle rides in the afternoons, the ritual games of backgammon after dinner. I tell her how we slept, his hand falling naturally on the back of my thigh, the gravity of that hand as I fell asleep, holding my body with a single touch.

We come to a stop at a clearing: a pasture ringed by shedding birches, a white-shingled farmhouse, a leaf-dotted stream. Light gleams from the trees. The place looks so familiar, but I know I've never been here before.

The next day Kristin and I drive through the New England towns, with their old churches and their candy shops. We drink apple cider and eat thick slabs of cheddar cheese. We visit a monastery where the monks pray by sitting in a circle, their sneakered feet side by side on the floor of an old barn—eyes closed, smiling. Some of the monks wear jeans under their chocolate-colored robes. They strum guitars and sing about a love simple and sustained—songs with melodic lines that rise and fall like the breath of someone in deep slumber.

We hike to the top of Shrewsbury Peak. I'm feeling strangely disappointed in this autumn foliage; I want the single tree that emits the radiance of a thousand trees shedding their leaves at once. At the top of the hill, a brutal wind tears at our jackets, our hands. But we sit in the shelter of a boulder to read poetry aloud—to each other, and to the trees laid out like a hooked rug at our feet.

Kristin goes first, holding a book of Mary Oliver poems like a Bible, her alto voice rising above the wind. As I listen, I realize it's the silence I crave in these poems, an emptiness that cushions each word: *Beyond. Foolish. Happiness.* The silence is what's important right now. "Is the soul solid, like iron?" I hear Kristin ask, "Or is it tender and breakable, like the wings of a moth in the beak of the owl?" She stops reading and gazes out across the fevered hills.

III.

As I lay in my childhood bed in Los Angeles, religiously following the step-by-step directions in the needlepoint kit, my mother seemed to be always washing dishes in the kitchen down the hall—the water constantly running, the clank of silverware in the sink. Where did so many dishes come from? I think she sensed I was a little ashamed in front of her; before I was rushed to the hospital, she was the one to find me collapsed in the bathroom, in such pain

I couldn't speak or cry out; she had seen me vomit; she'd seen my robe pulled askew across my legs as I fainted.

But every couple of hours the water in the kitchen ceased, I heard my mother's footsteps in the carpeted hall, saw her tiny figure in my doorway. "You need anything, sweetheart?" she asked. She didn't wear an apron, so her sweatshirt was always dotted with dishwater. She stood half-in, half-out of my bedroom until her maternal instincts overwhelmed her; then she slid onto my bed, her palm on my forehead, her eyes teary with concern.

I can't remember if we'd ever really talked about sex; we attended the mother/daughter lecture in the junior high auditorium called "The Joy of Being a Woman," but that was more about Kotex than it was about intimacy, and even then I could barely stand the embarrassment. Once, feeling bold, I'd asked her if she and my father had sex before they were married. "Oh, of course not," she answered, blushing, turning to fuss with pots and pans on the stove. "And you better not, either." As she sat with me on my bed, I wonder if she looked at me, her daughter, and couldn't help but imagine what I'd done, if my sexuality made her angry or sad or ashamed.

My mother never mentioned my young boyfriend. She barely mentioned the pregnancy. Instead, she admired the growing needlepoint, rubbed the bulky fabric between her fingers, talked about having it framed and mounted on the wall above my bed. She knew that sometimes only the simplest actions are feasible, and those are the ones that lead us out of illness and back into the world. So I pulled strands of thread through tiny holes until one day I was able to walk, and one day I was able to laugh, and one day I was able to cry. Recovery, it turned out, was inevitable.

IV.

I see a woman sitting on the back steps, in the sun. Her knees are drawn up against her chest; her chin rests in her hands. She stares intently at the back fence, so that she doesn't see, or even hear, the screen door opening, the man stepping onto the porch behind her. His hand touches the back of her neck, so gently, and the woman nods. Her eyes do not flicker. The words have already been said; this touch seals them. *I can't do this anymore. I'm sorry.*

The words already said. The light sharp and expectant. Life unfolding as a series of slick, overlapping planes, tilted first one way and then another. The man lingers a moment, then he turns and goes back into the house. These two people begin to misplace the selves they have formed over the years; they are fading. Family, and the possibilities of family. The tender weight of sex. The image of his face facing hers, one cheek pressed against the pillow. The woman sits on the porch a long time, until the sun disappears behind the garage, and the gnats swarm in a cloud above the honeysuckle.

V.

Kristin and I go to a party at a millionaire's house and we dance, our arms entwined. We eat roast pig and mashed potatoes and cornbread and brownies, our heads bent low over the round table, like feeding animals. At sunset, when the light illuminates the stained trees, I go outside and remember that needlepoint—the bulky hills, the smell of bandages, the chalky taste of painkiller in my throat.

I remember his hand touching the back of my thigh.

I remember the stitches—in and out, up and down, slanting first one way and then another.

VI.

One of my nurses was a Deadhead. She had long black hair that floated behind her as she walked from bed to bed. When she saw a Grateful Dead button on my hat in the closet, she soothed me with stories about Dead shows in the sixties, parties with Jerry Garcia and Bob Weir, days spent smoking marijuana with the roadies on the red bluffs above Boulder. She told me about synchronicity, how everything happens for reasons we can't even imagine. When she went off-shift I stared out my hospital window and imagined I was now destined to be a mother to *all* children, not just one or two in particular.

Keith often asked me if I would try in vitro fertilization, a question predicated on a series of "ifs": if we were married, if we had money, if we were still young. I still had my uterus, I still had my ovaries—all I really needed was that microsecond in between. "Do you *want* children?" he asked, as if the wanting were the easiest part, the least complex of the maneuvers we needed to negotiate in order to bear children together.

Funny how our lovers find the place we feel most wounded; maybe this is what it finally means to love: to probe that scarred flesh and not hate each other for it. I could have said yes; it would have been a partial truth, after all. Of course I *wanted* children, those replicas of myself, proof that I have lived, people I could love beyond reason. So I tried to imagine myself going to the in vitro clinic, my eggs sucked up through a long syringe, Keith's sperm dropped into a petri dish. I imagined the fertilized embryos implanted inside my body. I saw the surplus embryos hidden in the deep freeze, waiting. I imagined those embryos eventually swept away into a dumpster.

VII.

Kristin and I walk all over Vermont. *You did the right thing,* Kristin says. I pretend I'm not thinking about my lover or the last time we kissed; I'm not imagining the women he will kiss from now on, his mouth soft and pliant and forgiving.

I dream I'm driving a car over a mountainous road. I drive that car over a cliff. I dream a whole family bobs in the waves, little children held in their father's arms, an old woman floating serenely on her back. We all survive, and no one blames me for the accident.

VIII.

When I return home to Seattle I see the autumn I've been looking for: one blazing red tree in my path, framed by an arch of bright yellow branches. It's not so much that I see the tree, but that the tree appears to see me—those dipping branches, the winking leaves. A chime rings and is silent; I hear a carp splash once in the pond. The gardener who planted these maples is probably dead by now, but the trees are fertilized and watered and cultivated with tiny scissors—to create this perfect arch, the branches waving gently underneath. The scene looks completely accidental but, in fact, nothing is left to chance.

IX.

If I wake too early, at four or five in the morning, I turn and face the wall across the empty space of my bed. In the dark, that space still holds the shape of a man—a numinous outline of shoulders and hips. And I wonder: where do our prayers go? our faith? our moments of clarity? Do we finally reach an arrival point, tangible and obvious as a train station? But train stations are only facades after all, prefacing the chaos that lies behind them—the noisy streets, the muddle of pedestrians, the line of taxis waiting to take you somewhere else.

Late in the morning I watch my neighbors in their backyard: two women who wear rubber boots and gardening gloves. They're always raking the leaves around their chestnut tree, or merely standing, arms folded, gazing at the side of their house. Their voices come to me in muted fragments, but I think, by the easy way they pass each other at their tasks, that they must be happy. I watch them while I should be doing something else: writing, reading, making lunch. I know the women have seen me sometimes, at my attic window, a pale face staring out from behind the glass; when they catch me, I shift my eyes and pretend I'm admiring their yellow dahlias.

I don't remember if I ever finished that needlepoint. Perhaps I recovered before completely filling in the farmhouse, the valley, or the hills. I may have left it half-finished on the bed, warped at the edges and dingy with grime. Recovery was the only important thing, my mother told me without speaking about it. The rest of life—that would come later.

When my neighbors go inside, I focus my gaze on the pear tree in my garden which, even now, at the cusp of winter, still pushes out a handful of imperfectly pear-shaped fruits. A sheet of Japanese rice paper veils the upper windowpane; long ago there must have been women, kneeling on tatami mats, weaving gossamer threads together to form the translucent leaves. The paper is white, and fragile, and impossibly beautiful, held together by nothing but the attention of its maker.

The Names

I AM THE DAUGHTER OF SANDRA, the daughter of Beatrice, the daughter of Pearl.

We're sitting in a circle on the floor of my therapist's home in Seattle. It's a Victorian house, with wood floors covered in plush, handwoven rugs from Tibet. Tonight we're supposed to chant our matriarchal lineage, as far back as we know, and some of the women, I'm surprised to hear, seem to recall a genealogy so long that time begins to unravel: the names bring us into nineteenth-century bedrooms, fatal childbirths, days spent peeling potatoes, boiling stews, sewing napkins. *Emma, Constance, Marjorie, Ruby*: the darkness here is warped by flickering candles, the smell of sandalwood and silk. This exercise is supposed to give us a stronger sense of self, to help us remember we spring from a matrix of feminine competence to which we can claim birthright.

But I can remember only three women, and of those Pearl is questionable; she may have been my father's grandmother, but I keep her in the lineup because a list of only two matriarchs seems ridiculously short. I feel slightly foolish, as I do with all ritual, so I keep my eyes open and watch the faces of the women around me. Some of them chant with the lilt of incantation, their eyes closed in an expression close to sexual pleasure. These are the women who already know they are women, who wear fuchsia rayon dresses and crimp their long blond hair so it shimmers across bare shoulder blades. Others mumble the names, their voices barely above a whisper, their eyes, like mine, skirting the edges of the room.

I am the daughter of Sandra, the daughter of Beatrice, the daughter of Pearl. It's harder than I thought, this gesture of acknowledgment, to say out loud that I am truly made of these women, that I am of their bodies, their arthritic hands, their worried mouths. I've spent much of my adult life separating myself from heritage, from genealogy, from the prophecy inherent in my mother's and my grandmother's body. And now I'm being asked to attach myself to these women without reservation. I glance at the therapist, who looks back at me and smiles encouragingly. So as not to disappoint her, I close my eyes, I try to do this right. I say the names. They sound hollow, disconnected. I say them again.

I am the daughter of Sandra, the daughter of Beatrice, the daughter of Pearl.

Of the three names, Beatrice is the one I snag on: my mother's mother, a Russian Jew born in Brooklyn in 1904. I hardly knew her— my parents moved us from New Jersey to California when I was a month old. I saw her perhaps once every few years, at her small brownstone in the narrow streets of Brooklyn. The house, I remember, had a *mezuzah* below the front lintel, and a clothesline out back mirroring hundreds of clotheslines up and down the borough.

I see her now only in fragmented images, like the photographs of DeCarava, subdued black-and-white, my grandmother already moving purposefully outside the frames I construct to keep her in one place. I mostly see her from behind; I watch her in the small kitchen in Brooklyn, her broad back moving from sink to counter to stove as she folded stuffed cabbage. I see her hands, swollen and disembodied, giving me a quarter to buy a chocolate egg cream at the drugstore. Or I focus on her torso reclined uncomfortably against the easy chair in my brother's old bedroom, one hand resting on a cane, the other holding open a paperback novel.

But the most vivid fragment I have, the one I believe most accurate, is Beatrice's face at our kitchen table, studying her Scrabble rack, her blue gaze ticking back and forth. She reveals no flicker of luck or worry. She cajoles words out of the jumbled letters, her fingers rough in contrast to the smooth, reflective tiles. I can hear the intermittent click-click of the letters laid triumphantly against the board, the words taking shape, emerging into a constellation of sentences that make a perverted sense: *break heads behind the yard. seals lick hazily. iota turns around.* My grandmother always won, racking up points of thirty, forty, fifty and more; we, the progeny, sat around her at the kitchen table, glancing now and again at that inscrutable face as we laid down our paltry words.

I remember no moments unmediated between us, yet I felt a closeness to Beatrice inexplicable through proximity or reason. As a child I often thought of her, called up that face as I played in my California backyard and imagined her moving silent in her kitchen, gazing out her window and thinking of me. I ran in circles among the eucalyptus; she made *matzoh brie* while snow fell on the sooty streets. Now, as I say *Beatrice*, I imagine a March day in 1959, Cherry Hill, New Jersey. I see her face crossing my line of vision, a blur of blue eye. I hear my name in a high voice, feel my name wet against my cheek. Such a naming goes deep, deep into the body. Just so, in later years, I would be *Sweetheart, Honey, Baby,* and *Love,* those names murmured against my skin as if I were an infant again, returning to a body with no edge, a flesh without resistance, molded into the baby, the honey, the heart.

I am the daughter of Sandra, the daughter of Beatrice, the daughter of Pearl.

I'm working this summer as a secretary at Myriad Genetic Laboratories. Technicians in blue lab coats come and go from the labs; their job is to distill single strands of DNA from drops of blood, trying to find the defective gene that causes breast and ovarian cancers. They publish their results in graphs composed of oddly beautiful colors: magenta, turquoise, ocher.

I handle a hundred Patient Information Forms, on each of them a medical history:

Relationship: Mother.

Age at diagnosis: 38.

Site of cancer: Breast.

On some of these forms patients list as many as seventeen women in their families who have died of breast or ovarian cancers. These women want their genes tested for a specific genetic mutation that puts them at risk. There are no preventative measures, short of mastectomy, they can take once they know they're susceptible. But these women want to know what they're made of, so they provide a vial of blood. They wait in New York, in Heidelberg, in Oslo for the results.

One afternoon my boss, Beth, waves me into her office and, whispering, asks me to fill out a bogus form to accompany an already known sample. She wants to test the lab technicians for quality control. "They already know my handwriting," she says, pushing the form and a blue pen toward me on her desk. She tells me to make up a name, a date of birth, a family history.

I'm a good employee. I do what I'm told. I become Anna Morgan. I'm forty-two years old. I'm of Ashkenazi heritage, and my mother, my sister, my aunt, and my grandmother have all died of breast cancer. I create a new matriarchal lineage for myself, one that narrates a suffering I can barely imagine. My hand begins to shake a little, but I finish the form and, laughing, hand it to Beth. I return to my office and close the door. I need to think about this. I need to think about the bondage of blood, how the smallest particles of matter bypass volition and make us who we are.

My mother, too, unwittingly passed into my body an inheritance both microscopic and dangerous. It began with an appointment, in the fall of 1958, at a clinic in Camden, New Jersey. My mother, twenty-four years old and pregnant with her second child, was a little worried because she'd had a miscarriage with her last pregnancy. She left her small house in the suburb of Cherry Hill; she felt young and pretty, still a young girl, really, with her small waist, her flaring skirts. She knew she was pregnant because she couldn't smoke anymore—it made her sick, and she'd thrown out her last pack of Marlboro Golds.

I imagine she must have had to wait awhile in the outer office, thumbing through the outdated women's magazines, *McCall's* or *Redbook*, her lovely, pink-blushed fingernails glinting in the fluorescent light. She read recipes for hamburger, articles on bed-wetting, the ads for perfumes and lipstick.

She might or might not have seen the advertisements for the new drug DES, the ones that featured a healthy, delighted baby smiling at the viewer. The bold headline exclaimed: "REALLY?" and in smaller print: "Yes, DESplex to prevent miscarriage. Recommended for routine prophylaxis in *all* pregnancies." My mother might not have seen such an ad, but her doctor did. He read it in his journal of medicine, or he earmarked the pamphlets left him by the pharmaceutical rep. While glancing through my mother's medical history, he might have nodded to himself and made a single notation in her chart.

My mother's name was called. She went inside and put on the starched gown, perched herself on the edge of the table. She waited again, and this time there were no magazines to keep her occupied, only glass jars of cotton balls, beakers of tongue depressors, trays of gleaming steel implements she knew she shouldn't touch. She always did what she was told, followed all the rules. She was a good patient, wife, and mother.

When the obstetrician finally arrived, my mother would have closed her eyes and imagined herself anywhere else. She knew she mustn't say anything, mustn't ask too many questions. He was a busy man. The last time she asked questions at the end of the exam, he cleared his throat and muttered his answers so quickly she couldn't quite catch what he said. Now, he told her to sit up and she did, tugging the gown over her knees. He scribbled on a prescription pad, tore off a sheet, handed it to her. "That should do it," he said, clicking his ballpoint shut.

She got dressed and rode the elevator to the pharmacy on the first floor. I imagine she looked at the prescription, but the handwriting meant nothing to her. Vitamins, she supposed, to fortify her during this pregnancy. She would do whatever she had to do to save this baby from the malfunctions of her own body. She would follow doctor's orders.

My mother carried me to term, and when I was born, on March 1, 1959, I was a healthy, good-natured infant, 7 lbs. 12 oz., with eyes so large and dark people often stopped us on the streets to ogle me in my carriage.

Nothing at all seemed wrong with me. But twenty years later, as a young college student, I became pregnant twice in one year. Both times these embryos failed to squeeze through my fallopian tubes and so ended in the miscarriages, the rushed trips to the emergency room, the surgeries, the long recoveries. After the second operation, I woke from anesthesia to the sound of a ringing telephone at my bedside. I reached out a hand, lifted the receiver, heard my father's voice on the line. "What happened?" I asked, my voice a croak. As he spoke to me I reached down and felt the mass of bandages across my numb groin. He told me they had found an embryo in my right fallopian tube. He told me they'd cut the tube to extract it. I was still a child in many ways, and I don't know which was worse: the news itself, or hearing the news from my father's mouth. I wouldn't be pregnant again.

Years later, a young doctor asked me if my mother took DES while pregnant with me. He swiveled back and forth in his chair, the bearings squeaking, as he explained that my cervix showed the classic "cockscomb" configuration of DES daughters, a clear giveaway. I later learned that over five million pregnant women took the drug DES on doctor's orders between 1938 and 1971; it turns out the daughters of these women are more likely to develop rare cancers of the cervix and vagina. Deformities of their reproductive organs often make them infertile. My series of abnormal paps, the precancerous cells on my cervix, the ectopic pregnancies: all these could be explained by DES exposure. The doctor was surprised no one had mentioned this to me before, and as he put away the lab slides and the long swabs, he told me I must look after my body, my female body, more carefully than other women. "Do you understand?" he said, abruptly turning to face me, his eyes sharp as lasers on my own.

When I ask my mother about DES, she has no clear answer for me. "The doctors back then . . . ," she says, then trails off, too upset to speak. The irony of all this is not lost on us. I tended to see my infertility as an appropriate consequence for a girl who broke the rules; when I first learned I couldn't bear children, I'd gone to the Hebrew Bible and read about the barren women—Sarah, Rachel, Hannah—whose stories confirmed my fears. Infertility was a deliberate curse, an act of intention by a God who "closed up" the wombs of inadequate women. My mother, conversely, feels an abiding regret for playing by the rules, listening to authority and doing all she was told. Neither one of us is right. Neither one of us can fully understand the complexities involved in trying to understand our bodies, to unravel the legacies passed between mother and daughter, between grandmother and granddaughter, the invisible ropes that bind us.

In my office at Myriad Genetic Laboratories, people come in to use the copy machine, to retrieve pages from the printer, to make jokes about the weather. I walk down the hallway to the bathroom, passing the beautiful charts. Some prophesy cancer and some don't; I can't tell the difference. I trail my hand along the wall and shake off Anna Morgan and her inheritance. I become myself again: the daughter of Sandra, the daughter of Beatrice, the daughter of Pearl.

When Beatrice dies I'm somewhere on the road between Mendocino and Big Sur, traveling with my boyfriend to visit my parents in L.A. I call home from a pay phone outside our motel, and my father answers, his voice higher than usual, strained.

"I'm glad you called," he says. Trucks pass on Highway 1, making it difficult to hear him.

"Grandma Bea passed away," he says. "This morning. At your Aunt Barbara's house."

"Oh." My mouth goes dry and I suddenly can't speak, but my father covers for me, filling me in on the details. Aunt Barbara lives on Long Island. My parents are flying out right away; according to Jewish law the body must be buried as soon as possible.

"How's Mom?" I ask.

"She's okay. She's been expecting it."

"Should I come to the funeral?"

"No, don't feel as though you have to come. It's not necessary."

So I numbly agree that I don't have to go to New York. I hang up the phone. I go back to my motel room and tell my boyfriend, who obligingly holds me for a long time while I try to fall asleep. I tell him we had a special connection, Beatrice and I, and he nods, tells me that he knows. I hope to have a dream about her, as I've heard people do with relatives recently dead. But my sleep is fitful and dreamless.

The next morning we continue driving down the coast, neither of us speaking very much, and I think about one of the last times I saw Beatrice. She lay with a broken hip in Van Nuys Hospital, and I'd come to visit, alone, bearing a care package of chicken and rolls. I paused in the doorway of her hospital room; she was asleep, her eyes closed, her sparse white hair splayed against the oversize pillow. I went to her and touched her shoulder. She opened her eyes, and saw me.

"*Bubbele,*" she said, and smiled. Automatically, I rubbed her shoulders a little. "Oy, that feels nice," she sighed.

So I continued. I got up behind her on the bed and undid the ties on the back of her gown. The smell that rose from my grandmother's skin was an odor withheld in my childhood, so strong it became a taste on the back of my tongue: mothballs in a drawer of nylon scarves, the seltzer in glass bottles next to the Frigidaire, the powder called "White Shoulders" kept sacrosanct on the bureau. And beneath it, the smell of age and decline.

I slid my hands across the flesh between my grandmother's shoulder blades; I skirted a ragged bruise beneath her ribs; I squeezed the nubbled flesh of her upper arms. My hands looked tan, smooth, and young against her pale and mottled back. I could see the underside of her breast, the swell of her thigh, and I kept my hands moving, feeling for the knots of tension and regret. For once in my life, I did not turn back at the moment of most difficult intimacy.

Beatrice sighed. A woman in the bed by the window cried out in her sleep. A nurse looked in and left. When my hands tired, I held them for a moment on the top of my grandmother's head, in a self-conscious gesture of blessing.

I retied her gown. I sat back on the edge of her bed and looked into her eyes, saw a blue on the verge of fading away altogether.

She brought her hand to my face, touched me lightly on the cheek, as she must have done when I was an infant, and, as then, she murmured my name, spoke me into existence. *Brendadoll*, she called me, her voice thick with the New York of her childhood. *Shayneh punim*, she murmured, *pretty face*, and her already moist eyes filled with tears.

She kept her hand pressed tightly to my cheek, and I reached up to hold it there; I could feel the skeleton of her fingers, the rough underside of her palm. This gesture must have cost her great effort, must have invited a pain that radiated from her broken hip, her bruised ribs, her ebbing heart. But she looked at me without reproach or judgment. I stayed still as I could in her zone of focus, for the first time in my life knowing her—knowing my grandmother whose name, Beatrice, finally sounded lovely to me, sounded the way it must in Italian, with every vowel uttered softly in a lilting endearment of love. *Beatrice*, I find out years after she dies, means "one who brings joy." In the hospital, she pressed my face as if her hand could keep me from death, as if those fingers held a warding touch and would keep me safe forever.

A Dharma Name

This morning I'm going to receive my dharma name. I kneel in the zendo, amid the bowls of oranges and the sticks of incense burning in neat piles of ash. Orchids adorn the Buddha, and a few sprigs of lily and thyme. Many candles burn through the early-morning dark, gilding everyone in the circle with a golden hue. Last night our teachers, Arnie and Therese, asked who might want to formally receive the Buddhist precepts; in doing so we'd be given a name in return: a dharma name, a private name, one that might reveal in its syllables a true self that until this time remained hidden.

It was the name that did it for me, an incentive like the gifts they offer on public radio pledge drives. How could I refuse? All my life, it seems, I've been searching for a name that embodies me without distortion. My brothers called me Ben, and I toddled through my childhood this truncated self, becoming what my brothers wanted me to be: diminished, easy to play with, a ball thrown from one end of the yard to the other. I renamed myself Amanda when I was eight years old, lengthening myself into the undulations of three syllables, levitating myself from the gravity a fixed name imposes. In college, I was Little Raven, trying to speak in the native phonetics of birds. In Hebrew school, I'd been *Basha Leah*, a girl in another language, a girl with whom I might correspond, writing in the strange calligraphy of Judaism.

For this dharma name, we didn't have to take all five of the Buddhist precepts: only the ones we honestly felt we could keep. So last night, on a piece of scratch paper, I wrote out which vows I would take and why: the second precept, against stealing in favor of generosity; and the fourth precept, to speak the truth as clearly as one can. I feel a little wimpy: I took those two, really, because they seemed easier than the others, the only ones that required neither renunciation nor hardship. But the precepts are tricky; I know that to live my life in accord with even these two relatively simple vows will require a great deal of integrity, and perhaps even sacrifice.

All night I wondered what my new name might be, and I recalled the Buddhist appellations I know: True Seed; Vessel of Light; Perfect Knowledge. Thich Nhat Hanh, a Vietnamese monk, wrote a poem "Call Me By My True Names," and by this he means he is several, he is Whitman's multitudes. "Please call me by my true names," he writes, "so I can hear all my cries and laughter at once...." In the poem he becomes the starving child in Uganda, and the arms merchant selling weapons to Ugandan military; he becomes the twelve-year-old girl raped by pirates on a boat out of Cambodia, and he becomes the pirate who rapes her. By this roll call, he finds his true self revealed, an identity bound to that of all humanity.

In northern California, where I lived for many years, people changed their names quite frequently, shedding identities that seemed to bind them like ill-fitting clothes: there was Cypress and

Enchanté, Nighteagle, and someone who called himself *Am*. Sarah, at fourteen, renamed herself Strawberry. Marybeth, a good Catholic girl from Boston, renamed herself Rhea Green, a woman who now found herself kneeling, revering the first shoots of the potato, the tendrils of sweet peas and beans. When her son first emerged from her, in that round shack on the hill, I held him when a name did not yet contain him; I held him in the lightness, in this brief abeyance before he became the boy he would always be: Sean.

When I lost my two children, I realized afterward I'd forgotten to name them. They left so quickly after all, and everyone said no, they weren't children really, just small aggregates of cells. I didn't know I was grieving for children then. In the mornings I listened to the California rain as it pinned me to the bed, the sound of it gentle and steady, and felt only mild alarm that I could not move, could not eat, could hardly speak. At four weeks, each egg was barely fertilized; if the expulsions had not been so violent, the embryos might have passed through me without notice. But they grew big enough to hurt me, that must have meant something, I thought, as I listened to the endless rain. Lately I've imagined the two of them as brother and sister, a boy and a girl: I even dreamed about them once, twins named Ira and Isabelle.

This morning, I kneel in the predawn, in a line with five others who have decided to vow something, perhaps quite a lot, to receive a true name that might redeem them. And the names of my children return to me: Ira and Isabelle, Ira-and-Isabelle, like a chant, a mantra that might spur me toward enlightenment. My own names echo in my ears, multiple and confusing. I'm an impostor here, among the incense and the oranges. Can I really ever open my mouth without telling a lie? Can I really give and give without a thought of return?

But Arnie and Therese call me forward. I shuffle toward them on my knees. On either side of the aisle my sangha watches as I receive my name on pink parchment: *Kind Speech of the Source*, scripted in ink, stamped with a red seal. A name that speaks of incorruptible origins, clear thought, a pure land in which every shard is rendered harmless. It's a name I want desperately to be true. And my friends there, in the candlelight, in the downturned gaze of the golden Buddha, seem to think it is so: they murmur and nod their heads in assent.

Basha Leah

I.

IN PORTUGAL I WALK SLOWLY, like the old Portuguese men: hands crossed behind my back, head tilted forward, lips moving soundlessly around a few simple words. This posture comes naturally in a country wedded to patience, where the bark of the cork oak takes seven years to mature, and olives swell imperceptibly within their leaves. Food simmers a long time—kid stew, bread soup, roast lamb. Celtic dolmens rise slab-layered in fields hazy with lupine and poppies.

It's very late. I've drunk a lot of wine. I don't sense the cords that keep my body synchronized, only the sockets of my shoulders,

37

my fingers hooked on my wrist, the many bones of my feet articulating each step. I'm flimsy as a walking skeleton; a strong breeze might scatter me through the eucalyptus.

A few days ago, in a sixteenth-century church in Évora, I entered the "Chapel of the Bones." Skulls and ribs and femurs mortared the walls, the bones of 5,000 monks arranged in tangled, overlapping tiers. A yellow lightbulb burned in the dank ceiling. Two mummified corpses flanked the altar. A placard above the lintel read: *Nos ossos que aqui estamos, Pelos vossos esperamos.* "We bones here are waiting for yours. . . ." Visitors murmured all around me, but not in prayer; none of us knelt in front of that dark shrine. What kind of prayer, I wondered, does a person say in the presence of so many bodies, jumbled into mosaic, with no prospect of an orderly resurrection? A prayer of terror, I imagined, or an exclamation of baffled apology.

II.

On Shabbat, the observant Jew is given an extra soul, a *Neshama Yeterah* that descends from the tree of life. This ancillary soul enables a person to "celebrate with great joy, and even to eat more than he is capable of during the week." The Shabbat candles represent this spirit, and the woman of the house draws the flame toward her eyes three times to absorb the light.

In California, one rarely heard about such things. We grilled cheeseburgers on the barbecue, and bought thinly sliced ham at the deli, ate bacon with our eggs before going to Hebrew school. Occasionally we visited my grandparents in New York; they lived in a Brooklyn brownstone, descendants of Russian immigrants, and they murmured to each other in Yiddish in their tiny kitchen. They touched the *mezuzah* as they came and went from their house. When I watched my grandmother cooking knishes or stuffed cabbage, I imagined her in *babushka* and shawl, bending over the sacred flames while her husband and daughters gazed at her in admiration. So I assumed my mother must have, at some time, lit the Shabbat candles and waited for the *Neshama Yeterah* to flutter into her body like a white, flapping bird.

But when I ask my mother about this, she says no, she never did light the candles. "I didn't really understand," she says. "I thought the candles were lit only in memory of your parents, after they died." She remembers her mother performed a private ceremony at the kitchen counter every Friday evening, but didn't call for her daughters to join in the prayers. My grandfather worked nights, as a typesetter; he might have worked on Shabbat, doing whatever was necessary to feed his family in Brooklyn during the Depression, and so my grandmother stood there alone, in her apron, practicing those gestures that took just a few moments: the rasp of the match, the kindle of the wick, the sweep of the arms. She did this after the chicken had roasted, the potatoes had boiled, and the cooking flames were extinguished. But my mother, this American girl with red lips and cropped hair, was never tutored in the physical acts of this womanly ritual.

The *Neshama Yeterah* departs with great commotion on Saturday night. To revive from the Shabbat visitation, a person must sniff a bouquet of spices "meant to comfort and stimulate the ordinary, weekday soul which remains." The ordinary, weekday soul? Does he pace through the arteries and lungs, hands behind his back, finding fault with the liver, the imperfect workings of the heart? "Some cinnamon is all I get?" he mutters. "Some cloves?" In my family, the word *soul* was rarely mentioned, but my mother, and my grandmother, chanted the Jewish hymn, "eat, eat," as if they knew our ordinary, everyday souls were always hungry. As if they knew we had within us these little mouths constantly open, sharp beaks ravenous for chicken liver and brisket, *latkes* and pickles and rolls.

III.

Outside the spa town of Luso, in the Buçaco woods, in a monastery built by the Carmelite Monks, the shrine to Mary's breast flickers inside a tiny room. I open the cork door, sidle in sideways, and face a portrait of the sorrowful Mary who holds her naked breast between outstretched fingers, one drop of milk lingering on her nipple. The baby Jesus lies faceless in her arms, almost outside the frame, the lines of focus drawn to the exposed breast and the milk about to be spilled. Hundreds of wax breasts burn on a high table, and tucked among these candles are hundreds of children—faded Polaroids of infants in diapers, formal portraits of children with slicked back hair, stiff ruffles, and bow ties. The children's eyes, moist in the candlelight, peer out from among the breasts and the bowls of silver coins.

The tour guide describes the shrine in Portuguese, using his hands to make the universal symbol for breast. I catch the word *leite*; of course the milk is worshiped here, not the breast itself, that soft chalice of pleasure and duty. I want to ask: what are the words of the prayer? Is the prayer a prophylactic or a cure? But my language here is halting and ridiculous. Whispers linger in the alcove, *Por favor, Maria, Obrigado, Por favor.*

I want to kindle the wick on Mary's breast, but I don't know the proper way—how much money to drop in the bowl, or the posture and volume of prayer.

At home, in Seattle, I volunteer once a week on the infant ward at Children's Hospital. I hold babies for three hours, and during that time become nothing but a pair of arms, a beating heart, a core of heat. I'm not mindful of any prayer rising in me as we rock, only a wordless, off-key hum. Most of these children eat through a tube slid gently under the skin on the backs of their hands; pacifiers lie gummy on their small pillows as they sleep. I'm sure there's a chapel in the hospital where candles stutter, and a font of holy water drawn from the tap and blessed. Maybe a crucifix, but more likely secular stained glass illuminated by a wan bulb. Mary's breast will not be displayed, of course—the distance between these two places is measured in more than miles—but the succor of Mary's milk might be sought nonetheless.

It will be quiet. The quiet is what's necessary, I suppose, and an opportunity to face the direction where God might reside. I imagine there's always a few people in the chapel, their lips moving in various languages of prayer, including the tongue of grief.

IV.

Our synagogue was near the freeway in Van Nuys, California, and it looked like a single-story elementary school, with several cluttered bulletin boards, heavy plate-glass doors, gray carpet thin as felt. White candles flickered in the temple. The Torah was sheathed in purple velvet, and gold tassels dangled from the pointed rollers. Black letters, glossy and smooth as scars, rose from the surface of the violet mantle. When the rabbi, or a bar-mitzvah boy, brought the Torah through the congregation, cradling it in his arms, I kissed my fingers and darted out my hand to touch it, like the rest of the women.

In Hebrew school, we learned the greatest sin was to worship a false idol. "God is not a person," my teacher said, "but God is everywhere." The Torah, though we respected it, was not God. The alphabet, though it was a powerful tool, was not God. Abraham and Isaac and Moses were great men, not God. "God is everywhere," my teacher said. "Like the air." I learned about Exodus. I learned about Noah's ark. I learned about the Burning Bush. These miracles were played out by faceless figures smoothed onto the felt board. The twenty-two letters of the alphabet paraded like amiable cartoons across the top of the classroom wall, and I was called by my Hebrew name—*Basha Leah*, which over time was shortened to *Batya*. I preferred the elegance of *Basha Leah*, enfolded by lacy veils, while *Batya* turned me into a lumpy dullard, dressed in burlap, switching after the mules.

In the temple, the drone of the prayers rose in a voice close to anger from the men, nearer to anguish from the women, then ebbed into a muttered garble of tongues. I tried not to look too hard at the rabbi, lest I should worship him. I averted my eyes from the face of the cantor. I ended up staring at my feet, squished and aching in their snub-nosed shoes. My mother's hand fell like a feathery apology on the back of my neck, and I swayed uncomfortably in place. The ache in my feet rose through my body until it reached my eye sockets.

"I've had it to up here," my mother sometimes cried, her hand chopping the air like a salute at eye level, grief and frustration rising in her visible as water. In the synagogue, waters of boredom lapped through my body, pouring into every cavity, like a chase scene from

Get Smart. I imagined my soul as a miniature Max, scrambling away, climbing hand over hand up my spine to perch on the occipital ridge until the waters began to recede.

V.

There's another kind of soul that enters the body—a *dybbuk*, "one who cleaves." A *dybbuk* speaks in tongues, commits slander, possibly murder, using the body of a weak person as a convenient vehicle. If roused and defeated, this soul will drain out through the person's little toe.

The word *dybbuk* is in me, part of my innate vocabulary, though I don't know how. Perhaps from the murmured conversations of my relatives in Brooklyn and their neighbors, the women with the billowing housedresses and the fleshy upper arms. I was only an occasional visitor to these boroughs saturated with odors of mothballs and boiled chicken, soot and melted snow. I may have heard the Yiddish words in the exchanges between my paternal grandmother and the customers in her knitting shop; I blended into a wall of yarn, camouflaged by the many shades of brown, in a trance of boredom, as the women clustered near the cash register. "That one's a *golem*," they might say, nodding in the direction of a simple-minded man in the street. A *golem* meaning a zombie, a creature shaped from soil into human form, animated by the name of God slipped under the tongue. Or, "He's possessed of a *dybbuk*," they might whisper of a neighbor's child gone bad. They gossiped about *nebiches* and *schlemeils*, the bumbling fools who never quite got anything right, swindled from their money or parted from their families through ignorance or bad luck.

Sometimes I sat next to my grandfather after he woke in the afternoons, and he explained the transformation of hot lead into letters, the letters into words, the words into stories. I held my name, printed upside down and backward on a strip of heavy metal. My grandmothers pinched my cheek and called me *bubbele*. They cried "God Forbid!" to ward off any harm. On Passover I opened the front door and hollered for Elijah to come in; I watched the wineglass shake as the angel touched his lips to the Manishewitz. I closed my eyes in front of the Hanukkah candles and prayed, fervently, for roller skates.

VI.

In the central chapel of the Carmelite monastery in the Buçaco woods, dusty porcelain saints enact their deaths inside scratched glass cases. Above each case the haloed saint, calm and bene-dictory, gazes down on the lurid scene below: a small single bed, a man's legs twisting the bedclothes, his thin arms reaching out in desperation. The witnesses (a doctor called in the middle of the night? a maid, nauseated by the bloody cough of her master? a scribe, summoned to write the last words?) recoil from the bed in a scattered arc.

And the saint? Somehow he's beamed up and transformed into the overhanging portrait, the eyes half-closed, the halo pressing into place the immaculately combed hair. One finger touches his lips as if to hush the tormented figure below. His arms have flesh; the lips are moist; the background, lush and green.

We have our heaven, too, though I don't remember the mention of Paradise at Temple Ner Tamid. Paradise, I thought, was for the

Gentiles; when my Christian friends asked me if I would go to heaven, I sorrowfully shook my head no. They looked at each other, and then at me, touching my shoulder in sweet-natured commiseration. "We don't believe in Jesus," I said, my voice trailing off. I thought our religion was about food. It was about study, hard work, persecution, and grief. But I've since learned there is a Paradise for the Jews; it is, in fact, the Garden of Eden, where the Tree of Life grows dead center. "So huge is this tree that it would take five hundred years to pass from one side of its trunk to the other." We even have a hell: *Gehinnom*, where "malicious gossip is punished by hanging from one's tongue, and Balaam, who enticed the Israelites into sexual immorality, spends his time immersed in boiling semen." Of course, such things weren't mentioned when I was a child.

But my mother covered the mirrors with black cloth when her father died. She sat in mourning, with her mother, for seven days. She may have even spoken the Kaddish for twelve months, since my grandfather had no sons. Certainly she lit the Kaddish candle on Yom Kippur. But I was a child. I didn't listen, or I didn't understand, that the soul remains attached to the dead body for seven days, and takes twelve arduous months—ascending upward, flopping downward, cleaning itself in a river of fire—to enter Paradise. I didn't realize the soul needs our help, in the form of many and repeated prayers.

Before me now, a saint is dying in his rectangular case, on a narrow bed covered with a single woolen blanket. I surreptitiously cross myself, the way I've seen people do. The gesture, so delicate, touching the directional points of my body—my head, my heart, my two arms—seems far removed from the passion of Christ. It doesn't feel like a crucifix I inscribe on my body, but the points of a geometrically perfect circle. I curl one fist inside the other, and I kiss

my knuckles, I bow my head. I don't know if I'm praying. It feels
more like I'm talking to myself.

VII.

Swaying in prayer is "a reflection of the flickering light of the Jewish
soul . . . or it provides much-needed exercise for scholars who spend
most of their day sitting and studying." I get out my yoga mat; I
sway down into a forward bend and stay there a long time,
breathing, and then roll up, one vertebra on top of the other until I
stand perfectly straight, aligned. I think about moving a little, and I
do, like the oracle's pendulum that swings to and fro in answer to
an unspoken question.

VIII.

When I was sixteen, I became president of my Jewish youth group,
and we set out to create *meaningful* Shabbat ceremonies, feeding
each other *challah* on Friday night, reading passages from Rod
McKuen, holding hands in a circle and rapping about our
relationships. We petitioned for and received permission for a
slumber party, properly chaperoned by our counselors—college
students in their early twenties. The minutes from the planning
meetings illustrate our real concerns: "It was decided no one under
the age of twenty can sleep on the couches." "Challah will be split
equally before anyone begins to eat." "Ronnie says no wine. So
Mike's in charge of the grape juice." We rented spin-art machines.
We got a Ping-Pong table. We decided to give Ronnie a bar mitzvah.

Ronnie had a black mustache and dreamy brown eyes. He wore tight jeans and read Dylan Thomas. When he confessed that he'd never been bar mitzvahed, we clucked over him like a gaggle of grandmothers. We made plans in the bathroom. We took out every prayerbook we could find. We found him a yarmulke and a dingy tallis to drape across his shoulders. *"Baruch atah adonai,"* we chanted in unison, *"eloheinu, melech ha'olum...."* We closed our eyes, and the prayers trailed off when we didn't know the words; we moved our lips in the parched, desperate way of the old people in synagogue. We swayed back and forth; we felt mature, and very wise. Someone gave a speech enumerating all of Ronnie's strong points. Ronnie gave a speech telling us how he expected to improve in the coming years. We improvised a Torah with pillows, and we made him walk among us, beneath an arch made of our intertwined hands.

I think he cried then, his lips scrunched tight together, a Kleenex in his hand. I remember his thanks, and I remember us sitting in a circle around him, our eager hands damp with sweat, our satisfied faces aglow.

IX.

I call home from a post office in Lisbon. My booth, number four, is hot and dusty, my hands already clumsy with sweat, and I dial the many numbers I need to connect me with home. Like the Kabbalists, manipulating the letters of the alphabet, I work this dreary magic. Travel has not agreed with me. I have a fever, and I want to lie down, but my pension has a dark, steep staircase and soggy newspapers in the windows holding back the rain.

My mother answers the phone. I picture her at the kitchen counter: the long wall of photographs tacked together on a bulletin board—all the children, my two brothers and I, peering out at my mother from our many ages. She sits in the green vinyl chair, picking up her ballpoint to doodle. The lace *Shalom* hangs motionless in the entry. A red-clay menorah sits on the mantel, the candleholders shaped like chubby monks, their hands uplifted.

"How's everything?" I ask. We talk in a rush. "How are you?" she asks again and again. Not until I'm almost ready to hang up does she mention: "Well there is a little problem."

"What?"

"Everything's a little *meshuga*," she says, and her voice gets that catch; I can see her biting her lower lip, pushing her hand up into the hair at her forehead. "I'll put your father on," she says, and I hear the phone change hands.

"Your mother," he says.

"What?"

"Your mother had to have a hysterectomy. They found some cancer."

"What?"

"She's okay," my father says. "Everything's okay."

"A hysterectomy?"

"They got it all, the cancer. They found it early enough. Don't worry."

I'm breaking out in a damp sweat across my face, under my arms. I can't think of anything to say but, "Why didn't she tell me herself?"

"Don't worry," my father says. "Everything's fine."

I decide to believe him. After a few more distance-filled exchanges, our voices overlapping with the delay, I hang up. I push my way past the people waiting for my booth, I pay my *escudos*, I walk out on the *Avenida Da Liberdade* among the taxis and the busses. I start walking to the north, but I don't know where I'm going, so I turn around and head to the south along the busy, tree-lined boulevard. I stumble past the National Theater, past a vendor selling brass doorknockers the shape of a hand. What am I looking for? A synagogue? Or another shrine, this one to Mary's womb?

"In the womb a candle burns," the Kabbalah tells us, "the light of which enables the embryo to see from one end of the world to the other. One of the angels teaches it the Torah, but just before birth the angel touches the embryo on the top lip, so it forgets all it has learnt, hence the cleavage on a person's upper lip."

I want to light a candle, the flame sputtering in a bed of salt water and blood. If I had the lace scarf my grandmother gave me when she died, I might slip into a stone synagogue, cover my head, and follow the words of the Torah. But I don't know how. I don't know to whom I'd be praying; I thought we weren't allowed to worship a human God, so I eradicated the concept of God entirely. *It was all a mistake,* I want to say now. *I wasn't listening.* I don't know how to take the alphabet and assemble the letters into a prayer.

There is a Kabbalah tale about an illiterate man who merely uttered the Hebrew alphabet, trusting that God would turn the letters into the necessary words. His prayers, the story goes, were quite potent. But I can hardly remember the alphabet. *Alef, Gimmel, Chet....* I don't remember the Hebrew word for "please." I remember the words *Aba, Ima.* Father, Mother. I remember the letters tripping across the ceiling, the letters minus their vowels, invisible sounds we needed to learn by heart.

X.

A touch of the angel's finger, and knowledge ceases. I touch my lip, the cleavage. *Do you remember?* I ask myself. *Do you?* Something glimmers, like a stone worn an odd color under the stream, but my vision is clouded by a froth of rushing water. Perhaps knowledge exists in the amnion; the fluid is knowledge itself, and the angel's fingernail is sharp; his touch splits the sac, and drains us dumb.

The *mikveh* is a gathering of living waters—pure water from rain or a natural spring. This public bath was the center of any Jewish village; the water refined the body, washed off any unclean souls residing there. A woman stepping into these baths purified herself before marital relations with her husband; on emergence the first object she spied determined the kind of child she might conceive. If she saw a horse, this meant a happy child. A bird might equal spiritual beauty. If she saw an inauspicious omen—a dog, say, with its ugly tongue, or a swine—she could return to the bath and start again.

"The Talmud tells how Rabbi Yochanan, a Palestinian sage of handsome appearance, used to sit at the entrance to the *mikveh*, so that women would see him and have beautiful children like him. To those who questioned his behavior, he answered that he was not troubled by unchaste thoughts on seeing the women emerge, for to him they were like white swans."

What do I see when I step from my tub? My own body, lean and young in the mirror, kneeling to pull the plug and scrub the white porcelain. What do I see when I step from the baths of the Luso spa? Water arcing from the fountain, and all the Portuguese women gathered round its many spouts: bending forward, kneeling, holding out cups and jugs to be filled. A grandmother—in black scarf, wool skirt, and thick stockings—turns to me and smiles.

XI.

At my cousin Murray's house, brisket and matzoh balls and potato kugel lay heavy on the oak table. The curtains were drawn; I think of them as black, but they couldn't have been. They were probably maroon, and faintly ribbed like corduroy. I remember an easy chair; and my cousin in the easy chair looking too tense to be reclined; he should have been ramrod straight, the murmur of relatives lapping against him. My memory is hazy with the self-centered fog of childhood, the deep boredom, my eyes at table height, scanning the food.

"If only she'd gotten the dog," someone murmured, not to anyone in particular. This must have been a funeral. I remember my cousin Anita being "found." I didn't understand what that meant, but my cousins were sitting in the living room, covering their faces with their hands. Their yarmulkes slipped sideways off the crowns of their head. I remember the gesture, that's all—three grown men, slumped in chairs, their hands covering their eyes as if they couldn't bear to see any longer. As if they had already seen too much.

I don't think I went to the service. All I remember clearly is the food on the table: platters of chicken, congealing; baskets of knotted rolls; tureens of yellowish soup. And the men in the living room, so contorted in their grief. When I think of my cousins, I see them framed between the legs of adults, in a triangle of light, frozen. No one ate. All that food: for the extra souls, the one extra soul who wouldn't leave the room, even though the burial must have taken place according to Jewish Law, as soon as possible. Someone must have washed the body, anointed her with oil, wrapped her in a shroud. But a soul hovered in the corner of the room, a darkness smudging the corners of my vision. Eat, someone said, it is good to eat, and a plate was brought into my hands.

XII.

"One who cleaves." The definition of the word "cleave" is twofold and contradictory: to cleave means both to split apart and to adhere. Perhaps one is not possible without the other. Perhaps we need to break open before anything can enter us. Or maybe we have to split apart that to which we cling fast.

In yoga class, my teacher tells us to "move from the inner body." We glide our arms and our legs through a substance "thicker than air, like deep water." We swim through the postures. The Sphinx pose. Sun Salute. Tree. I generate intent before the muscles follow. I breathe deeply, I stretch sideways, I reach up, I bring my hands together at my heart. *Namasté*, I whisper. *Namasté*. I know my access to composure is through attention to the pathways and cavities of my body, so I sit cross-legged, my forehead bent to the ground in a posture of deep humility. Sometimes, then, I feel whatever *dybbuks* cling inside me loosen their hold; they begin the long slide down my skeleton to drain out through my little toe.

XIII.

I have a snapshot taken of me when I was eighteen. I've got long straight hair, and I'm wearing a Saint Christopher medal around my neck. It falls between my breasts. On another, shorter chain, I wear a gold "chai," the Hebrew letter for "life." It clings to the bare skin between my collarbones.

The medal was given to me by my first boyfriend—a boy I cleaved to, a boy by whom I was cleaved, split apart. I was *crazy* for him. I wanted the medal because I had seen it on his chest; I had gripped it in my fingers as we made love. He draped the pendant over my head, and kissed me between the eyes.

Eighteen years later, I still have Saint Christopher—a gnarled old man carrying a child on his shoulder, a knotted staff clutched in one hand. He dangles off the edge of my windowsill, next to a *yad* amulet inset with a stone from the Dead Sea. I have candles on the windowsill, their flames swaying to and fro, like little people in prayer.

A Catholic friend tells me that Saint Christopher is no longer a saint; the Vatican has declared him a nonentity. His life is now mere fable about the Christ child crossing a river on the ferryman's shoulders, growing so heavy he became the weight of every bird and tree and animal, the combined tonnage of mankind's suffering. But the ferryman, being a good man, kept at his task, his knees buckling, his back breaking, until he had safely ferried the small child to shore. "It's just a story," my friend says, but I don't understand how this tale differs from the other biblical accounts: the walking on water, the bread into body, the wine into blood. "It is different," my friend assures me. "Saint Christopher never existed."

But I know people still pray to him. They believe he intervenes in emergency landings, rough storms at sea, close calls on the freeway. Words of terror and belief form a presence too strong to be revoked. I still take him on the road; *It couldn't hurt,* as my grandmother used to say, with that small Jewish shrug, an arch of her plucked eyebrows. All this, whatever you call it—superstition, religion, mysticism—do what makes you happy, *bubbele.*

XIV.

Alef, Gimmel, Chet... I recite the letters I know, and they grow steady as an incantation, a continual flame. The Kabbalists manipulated the letters into the bodies of living animals and men. They know an alphabet behind the alphabet, a whisper that travels up the Tree of Life like water.

White swans. I dream I am wrapped only in a white sheet, and the Hasidic men turn their square shoulders against me; they will not touch me, they will not talk to me, because I am a woman. I am unclean and dangerous. If I do not follow the law—if I do not light the Sabbath lamp, if I touch the parchment of the Torah, if I look at a man while I'm menstruating—I will be punished by death in childbirth. Punished when I'm most vulnerable, during the act that makes me most a woman. But what about Miriam? I plead. What about Rachel, and Leah, and Ruth? They were women. They saved us. It is a woman who brings the Sabbath light into the home. It is a woman who resides as a divine spirit in the Wailing Wall. But the men, in their black coats, their black hats—the men turn away. They ignore me. I grip the white sheet tighter against me as the men file into the synagogue, muttering.

XV.

I'm staying in a pink mansion on a hill overlooking Luso. It used to be the residence of a countess, and the breakfast waitress makes fun of my halting Portuguese. *"Pequeno leite,"* I say in my submissive voice as she raises the pot of warm milk. I only want a little, but she drenches my coffee anyway, laughing.

In the evening I stroll down a winding street, past two women waiting at their windows, their wrinkled elbows resting on the sill. I don't know what they're waiting for: children to come home, or perhaps the pork to grow tender in the stew. They wave to me, amused. Another woman splashes bleach outside her doorway and kneels to scrub the already whitened stone. Bougainvillea, bright as blood, clings to her windowsill. Men are nowhere in sight; this appears to be a province maintained entirely by women. I make my way to a stone bridge and watch the sun sink beyond fields of flowering potatoes.

In the distance, women harvest vegetables in a field. I think they are women, but I can't be sure; all I see are the silhouettes of their bodies bending, and lifting, and bending again. These women—are they the ones who walk to the monastery and tuck pictures of their children between Mary's breasts? Do they pray before that altar? I don't know; they seem always to be working, or resting from their work.

Back in the square, the Portuguese men emerge to sit in clusters, wearing hats and wool vests; they walk down the lanes, their hands behind their backs, or they stand together, leaning on wooden canes. I sit on a bench facing the fountain, and the men converse around me, all inflection and vowels, grunts and assents. I'm silent as a hub, turned by words without meaning, without sense.

XVI.

The *luz* bone is a hub, unyielding. "An indestructible bone, shaped like an almond, at the base of the spine, around which a new body will be formed at the Resurrection of the Dead." The *luz* bone feeds only off the *melaveh malkah*, the meal eaten on Saturday night to break the Sabbath. It's a bone without sin, taking no part in Adam's gluttony in the garden; so, our new bodies on the day of judgment will be sweet and pure.

For proof of its durability, three men in a Jewish village tested a *luz* bone. (Like magpies, did they pluck the bone out of the rubble of an old man? or of a woman dead in childbirth? or of a child?) They smuggled the bone to the outskirts of their village, to a black-smith's shop, the fires glowing red in the stove. They thrust the vertebra in the coals; they plunged it under water; they beat upon it with sledgehammers. I can see them, these men dressed in ripe wool, sweating, their black hats tilted back on their heads. They hold it up to the light of the moon, the bone glossy from its trials, but intact. It's smooth as an egg, oval and warm.

XVII.

"...those who bow to God in prayer are thought to guarantee themselves a resurrected body, because they stimulate the *luz* bone when they bend their spine."

Downward-Facing Dog: the sit-bones lifted upward. Forward bend. Triangle. Warrior I, II, III. Sphinx. Cobra. Cow. These words come to me like directives, and my body twists and bends and turns, gyrating in a circle around the *luz* bone.

The Tree. I balance on one foot, the other pressed into my thigh. I put my hands together in front of my chest. I breathe. I look past my reflection in the window; I focus my gaze on the trunk of a holly. I grow steady and invisible. The alphabet hangs from my branches like oddly-shaped fruit.

Child's pose. I curl into a fetal position on the mat.

Nu? I hear my mother's voice across a great distance. *Nu, bubbele?* She pats one hand on her swollen abdomen, and holds it there. I want to answer, but from my mouth comes a watery language no one can understand.

Next Year in Jerusalem

Why is this night different from all other nights?

At Passover every year, I dipped the greens in salt water to remind me of my ancestors' tears, and I chewed on parsley to remind me life is bitter, and I raised my glass of grape juice and hollered "Next year in Jerusalem!," clinking my glass hard against my cousin Murray's. At Passover, no matter how much I've grown, I remain a clumsy girl in chiffon dress and opaque tights, sitting at the children's table, my stomach growling as my little brother asks a question. His voice is halting but already proud of the story for which he's responsible. I look at him with envy while I suck grape juice off my fingers.

Why tonight do we eat only matzoh?

My cousin Murray, a small man but imposing in his navy blue suit and graying beard, refers us to our texts, the *Haggadah,* which tells us the answers to these questions, but I've stopped listening.

We dip our pinkies in red wine and fingerprint the ten plagues onto the rim of our plates. What are they? Locusts swarming the fields, hail made of fire, days of total darkness, rivers turning to blood. Ho hum. I eye the roast egg, the *haroses*, the matzoh on the Seder plate. It's always dark in my cousin's house; what light there is seems reflected off the gold-foil inlay on the Passover dishes. My cousins smell of Brut and horseradish. I eye the roasted shank of a lamb, its blood the mark of the Chosen Ones. I watch Elijah's cup. I wait for the touch of the prophet's lips.

Why tonight do we eat bitter herbs?

The Seder goes on and on; the voices around me rinsed of meaning or sense. I chew on matzoh and *haroses*, imagining slaves' hands slapping mortar between the bricks, the heavy poles biting into their shoulders as they draw cartloads full of the stuff to the pyramids. Someone is talking about the Red Sea, and I think of Yul Brynner chasing the Hebrews in his chariot, leather straps around his biceps, his bare chest glistening. I think of Charlton Heston at the edge of a cliff, the frightened Hebrews clustered around his robes. The walls of the sea part, and the Chosen Ones gallop through, wild-eyed in fear and wonderment.

Why tonight do we dip them twice in salt water?

As I grew older, my grape juice changed to Manishewitz wine, and I murmured the prayers dutifully with the rest of my family. When I was twelve, my parents gave me a choice: I could spend another year in Hebrew school and get bat-mitzvahed, or quit Hebrew school right away. Our school was a stuffy classroom annexed to the synagogue, with tiny desks and battered chalkboards. Every Saturday, I sat in that room and chanted the

Hebrew alphabet, recited Hebrew phrases such as "Mother is making the bread," and heard the tired stories of Abraham and Isaac, Noah and his nameless wife, Moses and the golden calf.

Of course, I chose to quit the place, my freedom those mornings as miraculous to me as that of the slaves in the Sinai. But my brothers, being boys, underwent the coming-of-age ritual, and they received bags of *gelt*, gift certificates, trips to New York. They held the Torah cradled in their arms, paraded it through the aisles of the synagogue while we kissed our fingers to touch the velvet mantle.

After my brothers were officially men, the Passover Seder grew shorter and shorter—the four questions reduced to one, the matzoh on the table lying almost untouched as we snuck into the kitchen for bread and butter.

From Hebrew school I had a detailed picture of the old Jerusalem in mind: the stone walls, the arched gateways, biblical light streaming into rooms where wondrous and miraculous things happened. I imagined black-suited scholars hurrying toward the *yeshiva*, though I'd only seen such men from a distance, during my family's occasional visits back to the sooty neighborhoods of Brooklyn and Queens.

I left home and forgot about Passover most years, until the care package arrived from my mother: an orange box of egg matzoh, a sleeve of dry *mandelbrot*, a can of macaroons so sweet they made my teeth ache. I'd forgotten, I thought, those words spoken so many times during my childhood.

Next Year in Jerusalem!

The clink of the wine glasses. The open door for Elijah. The *afikomen* in its white cloth hidden somewhere behind the *Encyclopedia Britannica*. We watched *Yentl* and *Fiddler on the Roof*, the tinny klezmer music a soundtrack to our lives as Jews in America.

No one in my family had ever been to Israel. No one really wanted to go. We had reached our own Promised Land: the warm, enclosed cul-de-sacs of the San Fernando Valley, where we lived in our tract house with a Doughboy swimming pool in a spacious backyard. We lived among minor television stars (the "Jack" from the children's show *Jack in the Box*; the girl who teased Tony the Tiger on the Frosted Flakes commercial). We ate cheeseburgers from McDonald's, and brought home heavy, greasy boxes of chocolate-chip Danish from the kosher bakery.

I traveled to Europe when I was eighteen, tramping through England, France, Germany, and Italy for three months; when I returned home, my grandfather asked me about my travels. His eyes gleamed as I told him stories about drinking espresso on the Left Bank of the River Seine, and eating peaches big as grapefruit on the coast of Italy. Finally he said, "And Israel? Tell me about Israel." He sat back and folded his hands expectantly across his chest.

I told him I hadn't gone. His smile vanished. He sat forward and dismissed me by focusing his watery gaze on the far wall of the living room; there, a *Shalom!* mosaic faced the main entry, and a *mezuzah* nestled in the doorframe.

"How could she be so close," my grandfather murmured, "and not visit the land of our people?"

To get to Israel, I could have flown from Naples to Athens, perhaps ferried to Crete and then on to Tel Aviv, a distance of about 2,000 miles: hardly what a reasonable person would define as "close." But I bit back my automatic protests; even then, I knew the physical distance between Italy and Israel was not the issue. The point was that a good Jewish girl would have bypassed Europe altogether, avoided the topography of the holocaust, and found her way to the Promised Land unimpeded.

Why is this night different from all other nights?

On July 2, 1994, I crossed the River Jordan into the West Bank. I crossed in a Jordanian bus full of Palestinians with American passports. My boyfriend Keith and I had our names written in Arabic on a permission slip from the Jordanian Department of the Interior. The river itself was a muddy trickle I could barely see; wild reeds grew thick in the mud of its banks. Though I was a nonreligious Jew, I had still expected to feel *something* as I crossed into the Promised Land. I expected some twinge of recognition or arrival. Even more so because all through Syria and Jordan I'd been traveling on false papers: on my visa application I'd presented myself as a married Christian woman, a teacher of English. Keith had bought me a fake wedding band made of brass.

At the time, I did not recall the book of Exodus, recounted every year at Passover, my brother asking the four questions, the ten plagues, the angel of death, the parting of the Red Sea just a hundred miles to the south. I was afraid, as my ancestors must have been, but I was afraid of bombs and gunfire, not of Yul Brynner in his gaudy chariot. I was worried about the length of my dress, and the Syrian and Jordanian visas in my passport. Arafat had just visited Jericho for the first time in twenty-seven years, and the right-wing Jews in Jerusalem responded by breaking all the windows of the Arab-owned shops outside Damascus Gate.

My rayon dress clung to my damp thighs as an Israeli soldier boarded the bus. His hair was slicked back with mousse, and his khaki shirt hung open to the navel. He smelled, surprisingly, of Irish Spring. On his chest, a golden star of David swayed between his dog tags. "Passports!" he shouted, his voice cracking like an adolescent's.

I held mine out to him. He flipped through it, stopping on the page with the thick Syrian stamps. He looked at me, holding my passport just out of reach.

"How was Syria?" he asked.

Did he know I was Jewish? Did he expect a denunciation of the Arab countries, a declaration of fealty to Israel? Or was he flirting with me, just making small talk? The Palestinian woman in the window seat steadfastly looked the other way.

"Syria was great," I finally said, directing my words to his pendant.

He said nothing, but his lips curled up in what could be taken as a smile. He tossed my passport back into my lap and continued down the aisle of the bus. His rifle swung out as he turned, butting against my shoulder, leaving the tiniest of bruises.

In 1967, I had paraded through the schoolyard with my Jewish friends during the Six-Day War; we cheered Israel, our fists raised playfully in the air. Syria was the enemy—of Israel, of the United States, of the Jews. I confused the Syrians with the Nazis, all of them in uniform, with dogs, rounding up Jews as a preface to execution. When I heard the word "Syria"—with its sibilant "s," its insinuating lilt—I saw only three things: sand, barbed wire, and blood.

I was wrong, of course. Keith and I, in our wanderings through the Arab countries, had encountered nothing but hospitality and eager friendship. In Aleppo, Syria, the streets were lined with stalls selling green soap stacked like bricks, mounds of cardamom in open bins, amber jars of rose water and orange blossom oil. We drifted by vendors selling *schwarma*, with lamb roasting on giant spits. Men lounged in the doorways of their shops, sipping tea, or they tilted backward on straight-back chairs, rocking to the rhythm of the crowd. They waved and called to us, "Where from?"

We answered, hesitantly at first, "America," and the men cried, *Welcome!* They leapt to offer a chair, a spare tire, a piece of cardboard. *Please sit!* When we passed a baklava shop the owner frantically waved us in. We communicated with grins and a smattering of French. He gave us sweet pastry and fried eggplant and Cokes. His three young daughters popped inside, swirling around each other in pretty flowered dresses, their black hair bobbed short. They stopped when they saw us, eyes wary, but after conferring with their father they came to us and kissed our cheeks. Their lips were weightless as butterfly wings, and their eyes regarded me solemnly as I took each of their hands in mine.

It was a Friday, the holy day for the Muslims, and Keith and I went back into the streets, drawn by the staticky call of the muezzin. The women were dressed in their formal Friday attire—blinding white scarves edged with lace, jet-black robes, and black gloves. Heat waves rose off the broken gray asphalt, a surface that turned to smooth marble as we approached the Grand Mosque.

When we stepped into the courtyard, an old man angrily waved us into an antechamber. He plopped a heavy black robe over my shoulders, slapped up the hood on my head, demanded money from Keith, and shoved us out again. The black hood cut off my peripheral vision, so I teetered across the vast courtyard in a cocoon, my vision reduced to the patterns of white and gray tiles, squares within squares, leading to the central mosque.

Inside, thick Persian carpets cooled our feet, laid out in a tidy mosaic, greens flowing into reds into browns and maroon. Men and women crowded up against a grated window; they wiped the grate with their palms, then brushed themselves from head to toe, kissed their fingers, rocking back and forth in prayer. We inched inside the crowd and spied something the shape of a head, draped with a blue cloth. Prayers thrummed all around us.

"Welcome." A heavyset man with graying hair and a white mustache loomed over us, smiling. He shook our hands. "From where are you?" he asked. And then, waving one hand toward the pulpit, he smiled. "It is the head of Zachariah, the father of John the Baptist," he says. "A great prophet. Come, sit down."

Mehmet introduced us to his wife, a young woman with a face round as flatbread, hugging a curly-haired toddler to her hip. She smiled at us, but said nothing as we followed them outside, to a raised colonnade surrounding the courtyard. A commotion erupted by the eastern gate, and a wooden casket emerged high above a crowd, bobbing on its way toward the inner sanctum. Men in Western dress led the mob, running back and forth across the perimeter until the casket disappeared inside.

The minaret's loudspeaker emitted the soft buzz that prefaces an imminent call to prayer. From across the courtyard, the bent figure of the gatekeeper rushed toward us.

"Can we stay?" Keith asked Mehmet.

"Yes, of course. You are my guests."

The old man, furious, pushed in close to Mehmet, who spoke back to him in a low, growling murmur. Both of them shot glances in my direction, and Mehmet returned to us, shaking his head.

"You may stay, but your wife," he said, pointing to me, "must go sit with the women."

Of course I would go; I didn't mean to offend. I meandered along the edge of the courtyard, the wool cloak scratching my arms and the back of my neck, the desert light glaring off the gray tiles. Carefully smiling, I lifted my head. But only suspicious female faces regarded me from behind the pillars. As long as I had been with Keith, I realized, I was cloaked in Western privilege, but as I walked toward the women's section, looking for Mehmet's wife, I felt this privilege shearing off, bit by bit. With Keith I was a tourist, an object of curiosity. But alone, with neither a husband or a child to validate me, I became an unknown woman, possibly a prostitute, an unclean object, profane.

I saw Mehmet's wife hurrying toward me; she took me by the hand and led me to a colonnade at the rear of the courtyard, in the shade. She bustled me to her mat, amid hundreds of mats laid out side by side in a patchwork down the platform. The women sat cross-legged on the ground, leaning toward each other and talking, their white, green, or black scarves knotted tightly across their throats. When I sat with them, one of the women scooted away, mumbling *"Haram!"*

I would hear this word over and over in the next hour: *Haram*, with an admonitory weight on the second syllable. I later learned this word means "forbidden," but at the time I knew only that the women began to cluster around me, tugging the elbow-length sleeves of the cloak down to cover my wrists, pushing at stray hairs that wisped from my scarf, pulling the flap of the robe over my bare ankle. I came to understand: *I am forbidden.* Their hands touched me all over, patting me into place; under these hands I felt like a very small child, or a doll made of damp, still pliant, clay.

Even in my discomfort, I knew I felt only a bit of what these women endured all their lives: numerous hands pressing them into a posture of shame, submission, invisibility. If my family had been Orthodox Jews, I would have been molded the same way, shunted away from the men, bundled into a scarf, taught to keep my gaze fixed on the ground. The shame of being a woman, the dangerous sorcery of the body concealed: I would have learned these things had I been a devout follower of my own religion.

Finally the prayers began and the women turned their attention to the muezzin. At varying intervals they stood to pray, bowing from the waist, hands on knees, then kneeling on the mat, head to the ground, arms outstretched, then up again, over and over. I looked down the row and saw hundreds of women praying, their robes layered at the hips, wafting a vague scent of olive soap and laundered cotton.

Mehmet's wife, with a wave of her hand and a lift of her eyebrows, asked me to pray with her. But I shrugged and shook my head. Would it be more sacrilegious to mimic the movements of prayer, or to sit in a posture of respectful silence? "I don't know how to pray," I said in English, surprised to hear a catch in my voice. *Afwan,* I said. *Excuse me.* Sweat ran down my neck, across my abdomen. Some of the women finished early, rushing through the movements, and again they inched closer, touching me, pushing my hair back under the hood. *Haram,* they muttered, *Haram.*

On another cue, unheard, the women stood again. I saw men wandering in and out of the courtyard, some fanning themselves as they reclined near the door of the shrine. I stood up and saw, far across the courtyard, Keith laughing with Mehmet. What could they be discussing? Politics? Family? Food? I yearned to be with them, to be exempt from the rules of women, away from these women's hands. But Mehmet's wife pulled me back from the ledge. She again motioned, this time a little more forcefully, for me to pray.

So I did. I bent, placed my hands on my knees, and tried to feel something, anything resembling a prayer. I followed Mehmet's wife, moving my hands, my head, my lips. I hardly remembered praying in my own synagogue, mumbling along beside my mother and father, tired and hot and hungry, smelling the stale odors of mothballs and Emeraude, prune Danish and Folgers coffee. I remembered sitting at my Hebrew school desk while the teacher called the roll, and my own name—*Basha Leah*—ringing in my ears. *Basha Leah* drank from a sacred well. *Basha Leah* danced for the children. *Basha Leah* was cool and elegant, with wise eyes and a compassionate heart.

So, as *Basha Leah*, I prayed with Mehmet's wife—I straightened up, rocked a little on my heels, then sank to my knees and pressed my forehead to the ground. Here I could see nothing; the hood of my cloak shrouded me, blotted out the light. I faced Mecca, my arms outstretched, my head bowed in an attitude of respect and devotion. Millions of Muslims faced Mecca that same moment, sending the force of their worship in this direction, their prayers rolling over the slope of my Jewish back.

I don't know how long I stayed like this—face down, my back a shell, my eyes shut tight. But soon I heard the rustle and swish of robes, children querying their mothers for food. I sat up, my face flushed with heat. The women seemed to have forgotten me as they gathered up their mats and yelled for the children who chased each other among the pillars. A young man circulated through the women's section, selling sesame-studded bread from a stick. Mehmet's wife sat placidly next to me, her hands intertwined in her lap.

I wanted to tell Mehmet's wife I was Jewish. I also wanted to explain that I'd never been bat-mitzvahed; I was a Jewish girl, I would say, but I didn't feel like a Jewish woman. I wanted to tell her I could not bear children of my own, and so my future as a woman remained uncertain: how would I fit myself into a family history, into the traditions of my own religion? I thought she might raise her eyebrows, but she wouldn't grow angry; I thought she might smile and say something kind to me in a language we could both understand.

But I remained silent, and in silence we waited until Mehmet came to fetch us away.

Next Year in Jerusalem!

Keith and I pass through the gate into the old city of Jerusalem, inching our way through the crowded bazaar. There are dried apricots and peaches, huge bins of garbanzo beans, stacks of green soap, chunks of lamb smoking on spits. Boys careen down the steep alleyways with laden carts, braking by crushing their heels against a dangling rubber tire. We step over a threshold to the Jewish quarter.

The air clears; the crowd thins; spotless windows frame gold-chunk bracelets, silver amulets, hand-painted silk. The walls are a golden-hued sandstone; tract lighting glows from the ceiling. A gaggle of teen-aged girls swarms by us, followed by an escort, a man with a revolver bulging in his pocket. I see a woman browsing in a jewelry store; she's wearing a flowered-print dress, sandals, and an automatic rifle casually slung over her shoulder. A cluster of machine guns leans against a shop window; a tourist poses with an M-16 in front of a synagogue.

As if following a trail by memory, or instinct, we're drawn to a terrace overlooking the Wailing Wall. When I was a child in Hebrew school, they showed us black-and-white newspaper photos of Hasidic men davening against this wall, women crying, bar mitzvah boys hugging the Torah. My teachers spoke of the worshippers leaning so close to the stone they kissed it. The photos must have been snapped from exactly this angle: the Dome of the Rock rising in the background, and in the foreground the ruined gray wall, with its rough-cut stones and moss growing from between the cracks.

And, flush to the wall, the swaying line of worshippers. As a child I thought this was the place a Jew came when he was sad and needed to cry.

When my family held their wine glasses aloft and pledged *Next Year in Jerusalem!*, they had exactly this place in mind. The men saw themselves in tallis and yarmulkes, joining Jews from around the world in a steady chant. The women imagined rejoining their mothers and grandmothers in song. Jerusalem and the Wailing Wall were identical.

Keith and I pass through a police checkpoint and hurry down the steps into the courtyard. As if by instinct, I glance up at the rim of the wall for snipers. Two police vans glide into the enclosure; a cadre of soldiers clatters down the steps, and we blend into the crowd of tourists swarming toward the wall. On one side are the men, the dark mass of Hasidic Jews on the far left, rocking rhythmically; on the other side the women mill in muted dresses and scarves. A few people sit away from the wall in dull gray folding chairs, but most are packed shoulder to shoulder along the stones.

What am I to do, now that I'm here in the land of my grandfather's imagination? Keith leans down and whispers in my ear. "We'll meet up in a bit." He wanders to the men's side, and I see a gatekeeper drop a cardboard yarmulke onto his head.

A woman approaches me as I enter the women's section. "Are you Jewish?" she says. Her face is neutral, composed. "Yes," I say, "I'm Jewish." But the woman squints at me and continues her interrogation, unconvinced. "Is your mother Jewish?" she asks, her gaze roaming across my forehead, my nose, my mouth. "Yes, my mother is Jewish," I meekly reply. She smiles approvingly and hands me a blank slip of paper.

Then I see them—the prayers rolled up and stuck into cracks, falling in drifts at the foot of the wall. To my left, I hear the sing-song voices of the men, murmuring, and above that the occasional throaty calls of the black-hatted Hasids davening back and forth, their foreheads tapping the wall. The Hebrew sounds familiar as English, though I have no idea what it means. I watch the women on my side: their palms flat on the wall, their heads bent, their lips moving in mumbled devotion.

I've read the Wailing Wall is an ear to God, and that's why so many come to touch it, to press their lips against the mossy rocks. I watch the women reading sotto voce from their prayer books, or sometimes with no voice at all, just moving their lips and rocking back and forth on their heels. Eventually I get close enough to touch a tentative finger to the stone. This one brick is wider than my arms spread side-to-side; the surface buckles and curves. This was a stone laid down by King Herod's men, before the birth of Christ. It feels cool and comforting, and I would keep my hand there longer, but I back off quickly to allow a small woman in a gray scarf to take her desperate place at the wall.

From the men's section I hear one of the Hasids, his prayer warbling high above the muted voices, and one of the women next to me, her hands covering her eyes, cries out in response. I back away, as I see the other women have done, keeping the wall in sight. I've said no prayer, not even to myself; I've written no plea to the *Shekinah* who resides within the stones.

But even as I shuffle in humiliation away from the wall, I know on my last day in Jerusalem I'll feel compelled to revisit the courtyard alone. I'll take my place, leaning forward to touch my forehead against the wall. I might hold both palms flat against the rock. I'll smell moss and dust and the stone that still molders beneath the earth. I'll smell the breath of millions of women before me, and I'll smell the skin of the woman next to me, her lips moving, her eyes tightly closed. Prayer has an odor of devotion and righteousness, but here it's also the smell of milk and mothballs, scarves folded in a drawer, and seltzer for the grandchildren in big glass bottles next to the fridge. It's the sound of children fidgeting at the table as they listen to the stories over and over, chewing on matzoh and *haroses*. It's the sound of my mother dishing up the brisket, the roast chicken. I'll smell my grandmother, the powder behind her ears, and I'll hear my grandfather mumbling his prayer on the other side, a voice perilously close to song.

I don't know if I'll write anything down, commit my voice to a parchment scroll and leave it forever in one of the empty cracks. But I'll know how to pray. I'll turn my head slightly and press my ear to listen against the stone.

PART TWO

How to Meditate

Day 1

On arrival, huddle in the Volkswagen with your friends and eat all the chocolate in the car. Chocolate chips, old Kit-Kats, the tag-end of a Hershey Bar—do not discriminate. Feel deprived, then light up your last Sherman, pass it around. Watch your fellow retreatants flow into the meditation hall. Note how elegant they look, even in sweatpants and black Wellingtons. You'll wonder where they get such nice sweatpants. You'll look down at your baggy jeans, your dim T-shirt, and say, *I'm not dressed for this, let's go home.* Look beyond the meditation hall to the Navarro River, the cattails, the red-winged blackbirds. It will be raining, just a little.

Remember that you've forgotten dental floss. Take a deep drag off the cigarette and wonder what you're doing here. Take a close look at your companions in the car: your boyfriend Seth, who is so much older than you, and your friends John and Rhea. Remember how the four of you, just days earlier, had wound up tangled in a bed together, a soft bed with a down comforter, lazily stroking each other's limbs. Feel ashamed. Feel superior. Say, *Ready?*

A woman with bristled red hair leads you and Rhea to the women's dorm. There will be a deck overlooking a marsh where the blackbirds clack and whistle in the reeds. Glance at the other women who are folding their extra pairs of sweatpants, their Guatemalan sweaters. Sit on the cot and pat it with one hand. It will be hard, unyielding, to help you obey the precept against lying in "high, luxurious beds."

Scope out the meditation hall. Set up your pillow, your blankets, next to the woodstove near the back door. Figure this will be a prime spot—easy in, easy out—and smugly wonder why no one else has nabbed it. Realize your mistake when, during the first sitting period, heat blazes from the stove, frying the hair on your shins. Slide away a little, quietly as you can, and bump the knees of the woman next to you. Irritation rises from her like a wave. Start to apologize but choke yourself off mid-whisper.

Sit cross-legged on your pillow, your hands palm down on your knees. Breathe. Your teacher, who is from Burma, perches on a raised platform, his belly round, his knees hidden under his white robe. He speaks in a voice so deep it vibrates beneath your skin. He repeats the word: *equanimous, equanimous.* Invent a strange animal, an *Equanimous*, half-horse, half-dolphin, gliding through the murky sea of your unconscious. Feel where the breath enters and leaves your body just below the nostrils, like a fingertip tapping on your upper lip. Concentrate on this sensation. Within seconds find yourself thinking about Rhea's hand on your breast. Go back to your breath. Find yourself thinking about pancakes, eggs, bacon. Go back to your breath. Spend your first hour of meditation this way. They call it "monkey mind." Picture your brain swinging through the banana trees, its little hands clutching the vines. Go back to your breath.

Feel the pain begin in your knees, between your shoulder blades. Shift a little and feel the pain travel up your neck, down into your hips. Open your eyes halfway and surreptitiously glance at the meditators around you. They look perfectly still, their backs straight, their zafus round and plump. Look at your own flat pillow spilling from beneath your thighs.

You don't have the right equipment for this. You better leave now, before you're paralyzed.

Day 2

Read the rules again: No talking, no reading, no sex, no drugs, no eye contact. Vipassana, they say, is the art of looking deeply. Be unsure about how deeply you want to look. Read the schedule six times—4:00 a.m.: waking bell, 4:30–5:00: chanting in the hall, 5:00–6:00: sitting, 6:00–7:00: breakfast, 7:00–9:00: sitting, 11:00: lunch, more sitting, nap time, more sitting, tea at 4:00, no dinner, dharma talk at 7:00, more sitting. Add up the hours of meditation and come up with the number sixteen. Figure this must be a mistake and perform the calculations obsessively in your head, your own private mantra. You're already so hungry it's difficult to concentrate. Think longingly about the chocolate in the car, and hate yourself for not saving just a little.

Go to breakfast. Hold a simple white bowl in your two hands. Stand in line with your fellow retreatants and note the radiant colors of their shawls, their scarves, the blankets they have draped over their shoulders. Shuffle your way to the breakfast table. There will be large urns full of porridge. Take some. Take too much. Take a banana. Realize that your boyfriend Seth is opposite you at the table. Watch his hand as it chooses a pear, puts it back, takes an apple, puts it back. Feel a surge of love and annoyance. Out the corner of your eye see a glint of Rhea's blond hair. See a flash of John's denim shirt. Feel grateful and angry at the same time.

Sit down at the long picnic table and begin to eat your food. Realize you need some honey and scan the table, spying it at the far end. How do you ask for it without speaking? You decide to get up and fetch it yourself, to avoid making an embarrassing faux pas. When you stand up your knees hit the table, knocking over your neighbor's teacup. Irritation rises from her like a wave.

Go back to your room and lie down. Fall asleep. Hear bells ringing in the distance. Know that you are supposed to be somewhere, then sit bolt upright and run to the meditation hall. Slow to a casual walk when you approach the doors. Stand and listen to the silence a minute. Listen to the breathing. Open the door, which creaks on its hinges. Tiptoe to your seat, aware of everyone aware of you, of your every move. Settle in. Breathe. Fingertip. Nostril. Etc. Feel an overwhelming desire to run screaming from the meditation hall. Think about pizza. A cigarette. A beer. Feel your breath for one, maybe two seconds. Feel your neck slowly seizing up. Fantasize about yourself paralyzed. Imagine Seth and John and Rhea caring for you, running cool cloths across your forehead. Imagine the three of them kissing you all over your numb body, trying to restore feeling. Gasp when the bell rings. Hobble out the meditation hall.

Go to lunch. Hold a simple white bowl in your two hands. Shuffle forward and ladle yourself miso soup, rice, some wilted bok choy. Take too much. Reach for the tamari. Notice Seth watching you from the opposite side of the table and dab it on sparingly. Sit down and eat slowly, slowly. Wonder if there's dessert.

Day 3

When you wake up, you might hear two women whispering in the bathroom. If so, take the opportunity to feel superior. Calculate how long it's been since you've last eaten. Sixteen hours. This seems impossible. Wonder why everything adds up to sixteen.

Drape a blanket over your head and walk outside, toward the meditation hall. Notice the red-winged blackbirds, the budding lilac, the silver cast to the sky. You'll think it's beautiful. You'll think you'll have to get up earlier at home from now on. Pause for a moment and notice your breath, like a fingertip tapping on your upper lip.

When you enter the hall the chanting has already started. Your teacher seems to chant the word *Betamite* over and over, with variations in pitch and speed. Wonder what *Betamite* is. Think of it as a breakfast spread, sweet and salty at the same time. Think about breakfast. Calculate the amount of porridge you will ladle into your bowl. Top it with honey and a pear. Breathe. Notice yourself breathing. Notice yourself noticing yourself breathing. Your neighbor tips over, asleep, and wakes up with a stifled cry. Feel sympathetic. Smile a sympathetic smile to yourself.

In the afternoon take a walk down by the river. You do not have Wellingtons, so your feet get wet and cold. Your hands are freezing. You miss your friends. You feel alone in a way that is foreign to you. Try to remember if you've ever been so completely alone in your life, and realize how surrounded you've always been, how supported. Remember how you laughed in bed with Seth and John and Rhea. Remember the release of it, how it felt not so much like sex, but like love multiplied ten-fold.

Wonder if you'll ever be able to speak again. Try it. Open your mouth. Feel a tiny bit of panic tremble beneath your upper arm. Feel hunger in your belly like a wild animal.

Day 4

Just when you think you have it down, just when you've noticed yourself noticing your breathing for unbroken seconds at a time, your teacher tells you everything will change from now on. Now you must become aware of the sensations on the surface of your skin. Now you must scan your body, sweep your attention from head to toe, noticing the sensations arise and pass away. Arise and pass away. *Equanimous.*

Start with the top of your head. Feel your skull like a dumb shield, hard and unyielding. Feel nothing, then feel a slight tingling, a teardrop of sensation. Notice it. Move your attention like a scrim down the crown of your head, to the tips of your ears. Feel an overwhelming desire to run screaming from the meditation hall. Return to what you know. That fingertip. Settle in with the fingertip tapping on your upper lip. Feel competent. Feel sly.

Thirty minutes later open your eyes halfway and, without moving your head, try to see toward the men's side of the room. Move your gaze past young men with straight spines, men whose faces seem chiseled, calm, focused, unconcerned. Find among these men your boyfriend, Seth. See his furrowed brow, his downturned mouth, his clenched fists. See him trying so hard. Look past him for John. Try to find John anywhere in the room.

When you walk back to the dorm, see Rhea flossing her teeth on the deck. Stop behind a tree and watch her floss and floss, the movements of her hand so practiced, her teeth so white. Feel at a loss when she turns around and heads back inside, the deck now so empty.

At lunch, take the right amount of salad, half a baked yam, stir-fried snow peas with tofu. Hold your bowl in both hands as you find your seat at the picnic table. Sit in the same seat every day, though you could sit anywhere you like. Try to eat with chopsticks, the way the people in radiant scarves do. Drop bits of food all over the table. Try to brush them away, casually, with the back of your hand.

You've memorized fragments of the people around you: a hand, a wrist, a thigh. You know their shoes: Birkenstocks, rubber boots, thongs. You recognize their smells: rose water, underarms, unwashed wool. Feel at home in this. Then feel surrounded by bits of people disintegrating.

At night, you'll have trouble sleeping, though you're so tired you think you might go insane. Breathe in and out. *Equanimous. Equanimous.* Your teacher's voice is the only one you hear all day, and so you listen carefully to every word he says. At night, when you cannot sleep, briefly worry about brainwashing. Think of your brains heaped in a sink, rinsed repeatedly in cool water.

Day 5

At 5:00 A.M. you'll feel as though you're in a film. Drape your blanket over your head, clutch it closed at your throat, so you're cowled like a monk. Think of an appropriate soundtrack, something with gongs and birdsong. On your way to the meditation hall, you might see someone furtively smoking a cigarette. If so, feel superior. *Sweep* your attention from the top of your head to the bottoms of your toes. Make it to somewhere mid-torso before you begin craving kisses, wine, a cigarette.

After breakfast it's your turn for karma yoga, which means you have to wash the dishes. Stand at the sink with a man who, out the corner of your eye, looks incredibly handsome, radiant. He moves efficiently through the kitchen, drying the dishes you hand him with a rough towel. Imagine the two of you communicating without words as you plunge simple white bowl after simple white bowl into the hot water. Imagine you are married to him, that you have a house in the country with two dogs and a meditation room. Imagine the children you will have together, their terrible beauty. Feel him close by your side. He hands back a bowl you haven't washed properly; a gob of gray porridge clings to the rim. Feel as though you want to die.

Walk to the meditation hall in the rain. Think, *equanimous, equanimous*. Feel the water evaporate from your skin as you sweep your attention from the top of your head to the bottoms of your toes. Think about Rhea's hand on your breast, Seth's mouth on your lips, John's lips on your thigh. Try not to feel like a harlot. Try to remember how *natural* it all seemed at the time. Calculate how many different relationships must be nurtured in this foursome. Come up with the number sixteen.

At the dharma talk that evening, discover that you will now have periods of "strong sitting." Now you must not move a muscle, no matter how painful the sitting becomes. Practice "strong sitting" for a half hour before going to bed. As soon as you begin, feel an overwhelming urge to run screaming from the meditation hall. Feel a sharp pain radiate from your hip, your ankle. Resist the urge to move. Feel the tension in the room rise.

Then, inexplicably, feel your body relax. Feel the pain arise and pass away, arise and pass away, a continuous and fluid thing, impermanent. Begin to feel a glimmer of understanding. Begin to see your body in these terms, arising and passing away. Even the muscles. Even the hard bones. Even the core of you. Begin to wonder if the body that melted under the touch of Rhea's hand is the same body that now arises and passes away. Feel a bewildered sorrow. Return to your breath. Wait for the bell to ring.

Day 6

In the night, when you're not sleeping, have a terrible dream. Feel your body dissolve, turn into nothing but air. Not even air. Jerk yourself back. Lie there gasping for breath. Resist the urge to wake up Rhea, to lie down next to her, to feel her impermanent skin against your own.

Day 7

Decide to ask your teacher about this experience. You will go up to him during the question/answer session after the dharma talk. Spend all day worrying about this, about what exactly you will say, what words to use. Worry that your voice might sound harsh and ugly, like someone diseased.

Wait your turn. Kneel next to the stage, and know that Seth can see you, and Rhea. Try to look serene. John, you think, has stopped coming to the meditation hall, has decided to find enlightenment on his own. Bad boy. Envy him his initiative.

Move forward on your knees. Kneel before your teacher. His face is large, larger than your head. His eyes are kind but almost all pupil, and you feel yourself drawn into them, spiraling the way you did in your bed last night. So lean back a little, take a deep breath. His wife, next to him, smiles at you and you suddenly want to cry. Say, *I felt myself. . . .* Start again. Say, *I have so much fear. . . .*

He laughs. Fear is fear, he says, impermanent, passing away. He waves his hand in the air, and for a moment it seems to vanish in a flash of white. Thank him. Return to your place near the woodstove. Breathe. Feel the fingertip tapping on your upper lip.

In the last meditation period of the day, have another dream. Think of yourself pregnant, squatting behind a chair, giving birth to a baby girl. Feel yourself split open. Feel the beating of your heart, your blood.

Day 8

Breathe.

Arise.

Pass away.

Day 9

Begin to dread the breaking of Noble Silence. Begin to appreciate how much of your life is taken up with small talk and inconsequential matters. Swear you will get up earlier when you get home, you will speak only when necessary, you will be an equanimous person, even if you never touch Rhea or John or Seth again. Work hard at your meditation, so hard you break out in a sweat during "strong sitting." In the afternoon, realize that Rhea has been sitting behind you all along. Wonder how you missed her there, all this time. Before going to your seat, watch the back of her head, the set of her small shoulders. See her as a body already dead. See the flesh passing away until only a skeleton remains. Wonder how you will live your life from now on.

Begin to lift your head and look at your fellow retreatants. Notice that everyone seems a little worn down, pale, sallow. Look forward to washing your sweatpants, sleeping in your own bed. Wonder if you will be alone in that bed. Memorize a speech you will give to Seth, John, and Rhea. Swear you will love them no matter what happens.

Eat a pear for breakfast. Some rice and tofu for lunch. Steal some floss from Rhea while she's in the shower. Stop in your tracks at the whistle of a blackbird. Whistle back, a small sound made of nothing but air.

Day 10

Break the Noble Silence. Feel the buzz in the room. Everyone's giddy. You've all just returned from a trip to a foreign land; you all have pictures to show, stories to tell. Even the strangers look familiar to you. Say, *Don't I know you?* to everyone you meet. Notice the subtle glow around everyone's cheekbones. Sit with Seth and John and Rhea at a round table on the deck. Hear the blackbirds yukking it up in the glade.

Well, Rhea says, holding John's hand to her heart. *We've decided to have a baby!* A baby. The words seem so loud, so rough-hewn, you have trouble getting them from your ear to your brain. Rhea's gaze slides across your face. John looks straight at you and grins. Seth puts a hand on your shoulder, and takes it away again.

Forget the speech you were going to give. Start to tell them about the night you dissolved in your bed, about your fear of becoming no one, but halfway through sputter to a stop. Try to feel your breath like a fingertip tapping on your upper lip. Feel confused. Feel an overwhelming urge to run screaming from the dining hall.

Walk a path through wet grass down to the Navarro River. Say good-bye to the blackbirds and their red shoulders. Think you will always remember this, and know that you won't. Feel yourself rising and passing away, there by the river. Look upstream and then down. Feel yourself like a boulder in the middle, worn by the rushing water. Hug yourself. Feel your hands strong against your upper arms, holding yourself in place.

A Thousand Buddhas

My hand's the universe,
it can do anything.
—Shinkichi Takahashi

I.

I COULD TELL YOU I ONCE RECEIVED A MASSAGE from a blind person, but that would be a lie. I've never been touched by someone blind, but I can imagine what it would be like. She would read me like Braille, her fingertips hovering on the raised points of my flesh, then peel back the sheets of my skin, lay one finger on my quivering heart. We could beat like that, two hummingbirds, and become very still. Her hands might move across my abdomen, flick the scar below my belly button. My eyelids would flutter at her touch, and my skin dissolve into hot streams of tears.

I have never been touched by a blind person, but I have given whole massages with my eyes halfway closed, and the bodies I touched became something else. Their edges dissolved, and they spread out on the table—masses of flesh, all the borders gone. I touched them in tender places: under the cheekbones, between the toes, along the high arching curves of their feet. When I opened my eyes these people coalesced into something human, but I walked outside and slipped into the pool, feeling like a primordial fish, all my substance gone. I'd see them afterward, and they leaned toward me, their mouths open, but they hardly spoke. My arms opened and they fell against me; I held my hands on the middle of their backs, holding their hearts in place.

Sometimes they cried. I was too professional, then, to cry, knew that I had to keep some distance in order to make this relationship work. If I had cried, then we might have been lovers, and that would make it wrong somehow when they handed me the check for thirty dollars. Sometimes they pressed it into my hands and looked away, said *I can't even tell you.* I nudged them in the direction of the baths, and they went like obedient children, their naked bodies swaying under their towels as they shuffled across the old, wooden bridge.

II.

I have a picture from that time—of myself in the hot tub at Orr Hot Springs. At least, some people claim it is me, pointing out the slope of my breasts, the flare of my hips, the circumference of my thighs. Positive identification is impossible since the woman in the picture cradles her face in her hands.

Light streams through a low doorway into the gazebo, and this young woman leans her back against the deck. The sunlight zeroes into a circle on her belly. Jasmine bush and bamboo are reflected in the glass. The woman bends her head and covers her eyes as if she were about to weep. Steam rises in flurries and beads on the glass, obscuring detail and memory.

The woman is not weeping. She is scooping up the water from the tub and splashing it to her face. If this woman is me, she is mumbling some kind of grateful prayer, alchemizing the water into a potion that will heal.

It's easy to know what we're doing, once we're not doing it anymore.

III.

Before I lived at Orr Hot Springs, I spent a summer baking bread for fifty children on a farm outside Willits. I didn't know I was in practice for becoming a massage therapist, but I knew I mended wounds buried deep inside me as I handled the huge mounds of dough. The repetitive motions of my hands—the grasping and pushing, the bend of my waist, the slow ache in my shoulder—before long, I became automatic and blank. I kept my hands covered in flour and thought continually of food, of what is nourishing. I dreamed of my mouth always open and filled.

Children clustered around me, tugged at my apron, took little balls of dough and rolled them lightly between their teeth. The bread rose and came out of the oven, broke into tender crumbs, tasted good. I watched the children and gave them small lumps of dough to press. I touched their miniature shoulders and smiled, but said very little. At the midsummer dance, they braided flowers into my hair and held my hands, as if I were an old person convalescing from a long, wasting illness.

IV.

Today I look at my hands. I remember the bodies I touched, the lives that came through them. I look at my hands sometimes and trace the edges of my fingers, like children do in kindergarten on newsprint with green tempera paint. Hands become what they have held; our hands shape themselves around what they hold most dear, or what has made an impression, or what we press on others.

My friend Dana once grabbed my hand off the stick shift as I drove through L.A. "These," he said, running a fingertip around my palm, "are healing hands."

I drove with my left hand on the wheel, while he examined every finger of my right. I swerved to avoid a dog.

"They're like a sculptor's hands," he said dreamily, dropping my hand and gripping his own.

Dana is a sculptor, with a propensity for twisted nude forms, estranged limbs, fingers in a bowl. Once, he left for Ecuador and painted all his walls, the appliances, even his books, a startling white; a "blank canvas," he said, for his friends to spill upon. And we did, troweling up purples and reds, oranges and blues, a cacophony of personalities rolling across his walls.

I pressed my hands in blue paint and hand-walked an awkward bridge above his couch.

V.

What follows may, or may not, be true:

My ex-lover Jon stepped inside and closed the door, settled himself carefully on the edge of my massage table. "I just came to soak in the baths, decided to get a massage on the spur of the moment," he said. "I didn't know it was you."

We stared at each other. I don't know what he saw in my face— a barrier perhaps, a careful retreat—but in his face I saw a deep sorrow. My eyes involuntarily shifted into professional gear, scanning his body, making notes: a slump in the left shoulder, a grim tightness in the left arm and fist, chest slightly concave, breathing shallow.

In massage school, before we were lovers, Jon and I had been partners. The teacher insisted on partner rotation, but somehow Jon and I ended up together more times than not. We learned well on each other. We breathed freely; we allowed each other's hands to cup the muscles and slide so slowly down the length of connecting fibers and tissue; we allowed thumbs to probe deep into the knots. It was like a dance, the way our teacher said it always should be, an effortless give and take, back and forth, with the breath as well as the body. Communication—transcendent and absolute.

"Listen," Jon was saying. "I understand if you don't want to do this." His body leaned toward me, and I tipped forward in response. A massage room is a very close environment. Intimacy is immediate; truth prevails.

I glanced away from him and gazed at the far wall, at the painting of A Thousand Buddhas Jon had given me as a graduation present. For the last year, I had looked at that picture every day, and every day it reminded me of Jon less and less. A process of pain, moving ahead on its own momentum. The primary Buddha sat in the center, immovable, surrounded by a helix of Buddhas that spun around and around.

My palms relaxed, a good sign. "It might be awkward," I said, "but I'll try." I took a deep breath and whatever had been prickling at my throat subsided.

What did my body feel when I placed my hands on Jon's back? My palms curved instinctively to the crook of his shoulders; my own shoulders softened and I asked Jon to breathe, and he did, and I inhaled with him, stretching my lungs, and on the exhale my hands slid down his back, kneading the muscles on the downward slide, pulling up along the lats, crossing over his spine, and again, and again, until he seemed to flatten, and there was no distinction between the flesh of his back or the bones in his arms or the curve of his buttocks—no distinction in fact between his breath and mine. I felt a small opening in my heart, a valve releasing, and an old love, a love aged and smooth as wine, flowed down my arms and onto Jon's skin. I knew, then, that sometime in the night I would remember this gushing, and I would be shattered by a sense of tremendous loss, a grasping ache in my palms, and I would cry, but even this certainty could not stop my hands in their circular route through Jon's familiar and beautiful body. He inhaled and began to sob. The tears shuddered through his back, his arms, his legs, and I felt them empty from him in one bountiful wave. My right hand floated to rest on his sacrum. My left hand brushed the air above his head in long, sweeping arcs.

There is a powder that covers the heart, a sifting of particles fine as talc. It is protection—gauzy and insubstantial, but protection nonetheless. Occasionally, a hand rubs against you and wipes a patch clear.

That's when the heart bulges, beating with a raw and healthy ferocity.

VI.

There is another picture, one that is hidden in a drawer. It is me, before I moved to Orr Springs; me, before I even knew such places existed. I am young, young, young.

I am standing barefoot on the porch of a forest service cabin in Prairie Creek State Park on the north coast of California. It is late summer. I am wearing a purple tank top, tight Levis, and a forest ranger's hat. The morning sun is full in my face, and I am smiling a goofy, lopsided grin, my hands at my sides, my feet planted solidly on the wooden planks.

In this picture, I'm pregnant.

The pregnancy will end one week later, but in the picture I don't know this. I don't even know I am pregnant. I'm twenty years old and healthy from a long summer in Wyoming. It is a beautiful morning, and I am happy to be back in California. My world has not yet shifted to include the hands of nurses, the blind lights of an operating dome, the smell of bandages steeped in antiseptics and blood.

Look carefully at the belly for some sign of the child, at the face for some indication of motherhood. There is none; the snapshot is flat and ordinary: a young woman on vacation, nothing more. But I look at this photo and sense a swelling in my pelvis, a fullness in my breasts. I feel my skin inviolate and smooth, the substance of everything I've lost and meant to regain.

VII.

Someone called them midwife's hands. A midwife's hands cradle and protect, hold a life between them. The classic posture for the hands in photographs you see: one hand cupped under the baby's emerging head, the other lightly curled on the baby's crown.

There is a polarity position like this: at the client's head, cradling, not pulling but imparting the sense of emergence just the same. If you stay long enough, motionless, the head appears to become larger; it grows and trembles. Sometimes I have touched the top of my head to the top of my client's head, and we are plugged in; we take big breaths, heave long, important sighs.

VIII.

Sean was born. Not from my body. From Rhea's. I held the mirror at an angle so she could see the crown of his head as it split her body in two.

The midwife placed one hand on the skull and rotated it so the face pointed toward heaven. The eyes were open, glazed with an unearthly shine.

Rhea screamed. The world paused and listened. The body followed, sheathed in cream and wax.

IX.

What does the body hold? And how do the hands release it? In the late seventies, "hug clinics" opened on college campuses in California. Distraught people were invited to drop in if they needed to be held in place by a pair of strong, encircling arms.

One of the most powerful massage holds I've used has the client on his side, curled into a fetal position. I cupped one hand to the base of the spine, the other lay flat on the back between the shoulder blades. These are the two places our mothers' hands fell when holding us as babies.

Some people cried with little shoulder-shaking sobs. Others fell promptly asleep. Most of them believed my hands were still on them long after I'd walked away.

X.

In the hospital, the nurse pushed an i.v. needle into the back of my hand, over and over. I squinted and clenched my teeth.

"Does that hurt?" the nurse said, looking up.

I nodded.

"It's not supposed to hurt," she said, and set that needle aside, tried again.

When she was done, I lay on top of the covers, shivering, my eyes halfway closed, my palm flat on the bed. The i.v. fluid ticked into my blood. Already, I could feel myself forgetting everything.

My body was a container of pain. And then it contained nothing. An absence so absolute I couldn't even cry.

XI.

The hand is shaped to touch the different parts of the world. We hurt, and the hand reaches to the chest. A newborn's head fits snugly into the center of a palm. Fertile soil runs through our fingers, or we mold our hands into a cup sealed for a drink of water. We can use our hands like primeval jaws to pluck whatever is ripe.

The midwife had fingers so long I almost asked her if she played the piano. The words were nearly out of my mouth, but then she handed Sean to me, and I forgot about pianos, about that kind of music.

I held him while the midwife and Rhea struggled with the afterbirth. I held him against my shoulder. His eyes were open; he blinked slowly and rarely, like a baby owl. The light in the room was gold, the color of honey.

I thought I saw something in his eyes, but I can't be sure. I thought I saw a nod of acceptance, a little man bowing to me, his hands pressed together in an attitude of prayer.

XII.

They came to me hot and pink from the baths, most of my work already done. They came naked and slick and gorgeous.

What did I give them? Nothing but myself, and not even that, but the benefit of my whole attention, the focus of my hands on them, the focus of my heart. I don't know how long the change lasted. They left the room and lingered in the baths, got out, got dressed, and drove the two-and-a-half hours home. I waved good-bye and walked up the steps to my cabin, looked out my window to the woods, and thought about these people more than I probably should have. When the time approached for me to leave Orr Springs, I thought about them with a frantic longing for a life that could be balanced and whole.

I wanted to massage myself before I left; I wanted to send myself off with a stroke of my fingers, a hand along my spine, an affirmation for abundance, a momentary release from every memory that weighed me down. I thought it might help, if only for the drive out on the rutted and dusty road.

XIII.

Years after I left Orr Springs, I worked for the Human Resource Council in Missoula, Montana. I didn't massage people anymore. I tried, but I zipped through the parts of the body as if I were taking inventory. I chattered like a barber giving a haircut. I thought about dinner, gas mileage, bills to be paid.

In my job, I interviewed clients and determined their eligibility for a heating assistance program. Many of the people I saw were elderly and disabled; all of them had stories to tell, stories that could take a lifetime. I had only twenty minutes to spend with each one. I found that when I gave them my whole and complete attention for even five minutes, that was enough. I looked them in the eyes and smiled, laughed with them, murmured consolations. They looked back and told me what they knew. My hands kept very still on my desk.

One seventy-six-year-old woman spoke to me in short, disjointed sentences, her head nodding emphatically with each word, spittle forming at the corners of her mouth. She smelled of cigarettes and bitter lemons. As I walked her to the door of my office, she swirled around and grabbed me by the waist. I settled my arms onto her shoulders. We stood like that for a few seconds under the fluorescent lights, the computers humming around us. I slid one hand down her back and held her there; my hand quivered, near as it was to her old and fragile heart.

XIV.

I'm lying on my massage table. It's for sale. I'm lying on it, and I feel utterly relaxed. My breath swirls through my body in a contented daze.

I'm lying on my back. I open my eyes, and I see my face. I see me leaning over the table. My right hand comes to rest on my womb; my left hand hovers over my throat.

Forgive me. Those are the words that pass between us.

Sean Falling

A BED BIG ENOUGH FOR FOUR—the lack of such a bed became our focus and our downfall. Seth's bed, a queen-size piece of industrial foam, was wide enough but smelled of mold. John's bed was a double futon, battered and hard. I didn't own a bed. So most often we climbed to Rhea's loft: a platform soft and thick with down comforters, flannel sheets, and extra pillows. It might have been perfect, but the ladder was steep and precarious, and we constantly hit our heads on the rafters. The railing, built by the previous owner, was wide-slatted and useless; if one of us rolled too carelessly it meant a quick, painful fall to the kitchen floor. Seth and John alternated sleeping on the outside, their arms and legs hanging over the edge, while Rhea and I huddled in the middle, our breasts rising together in an offbeat rhythm as we drifted in and out of sleep.

Later, much later, the baby would fall from that loft. It was after we'd called it quits. After too many bruising nights, when the cries of love on one side of the bed transmuted to moans of despair at the other. I used to think love multiplied would equal more love, but it didn't work out that way. Someone always wept out of sight. The mathematics alone were enough to do us in. There was the relationship between me and Seth, and the one between me and John, and Seth and Rhea, and Rhea and me, and Rhea and Seth and me... the list went on and on.

We went to a couples workshop in a geodesic dome in Laytonville. The leader blindfolded all the participants, asked us to wander into the center of the room. We groped for the hands of strangers, then sat down and whispered our secrets. We unveiled our eyes, blushed, and returned to our respective seats. After the song of invocation, the leader asked us to turn and look into our partner's eyes. After much embarrassed shuffling, we left when we realized you can't look into three pairs of eyes at once.

Rhea's pregnant belly grew and grew, demanding more bunk-space. Our inability to find a comfortable bed became symbolic of our most intimate failures, so, in a gesture of resigned conciliation, we divvied into orthodox twosomes.

Mornings, Seth sat facing a wall and meditated, his eyes tightly shut, his throat taut and ropy as a turtle's. I drank coffee and watched him, memorizing the pattern of hair on the back of his neck, the lopsided whorl swooping up into a blunt-cut cowlick. I felt like someone named Tanya, in a Romanian village, learning to love the husband with whom I was arranged. When we made love, Seth stroked the hair away from my face and tried to gaze into my eyes, but his focus landed somewhere on my left cheek. I burrowed my fingers in the thick fur of his beard, trying to reach skin or bone. On my twenty-fourth birthday, he made me carob pancakes with canned apricots on top. *I love you,* I said, emphatically, but it was like mumbling the phrase to my mother on the phone—a farewell with a question mark at the end. He stared at his pancakes, apricot syrup congealing in amber pools.

John ambled over sometimes and sat at my kitchen table, chin cupped in hand, his long face moony. Alone, we'd twine our feet together, silent and excited, but nothing happened, nothing at all. We were good. We reminisced about the old days. John always looked like a puppy dog to me, the tip of his tongue resting in the corner of his mouth. Once he read my Tarot cards and told me I was destined to have many children, in a figurative sense; my layout was full of cups overflowing, and large women on thrones, their hands lifted in signs of blessing. He asked me if I loved him best of all. I told him yes. Seth asked me if I loved him best of all. I told him yes. Rhea wandered the pathway between our houses, her swollen belly leading, her face never losing the clarity beautiful women sometimes have: a glow having nothing to do with her blue eyes, her sharp chin, her pink lips, but rather with how these features merged—a continuous magic act—into one exquisite whole. I followed her to the garden, to the greenhouse, to the well. I did whatever she asked. I cupped my hand lightly over her womb and said hello to the baby as he kicked against my palm.

One evening, in their house up the road, Rhea threw a steel-bristled hairbrush at John. It missed and shattered a windowpane. Rhea fled into the woods and did not return. After dark, we heard a scream, oblong and sharp as a screech owl's; we gathered flashlights and water and set out along the river. We found Rhea wandering the road beyond the redwoods, her hands deep in her pockets, her white hair glinting at the moon. She looked startled at the sight of us, this squadron of concern. *Oh,* she said, *could you hear me?* Her winter coat bulged at the abdomen, wrinkled and stained. The four of us returned via a narrow trail, single file, Rhea in the lead, our hands linked together like a chain. Albino deer lived in those hills, folks said, and wild boar, turkeys, and quail. We watched for a flash of a white rump, an ivory tusk, a spotted feather.

Soon there was a baby in Rhea's house, and I napped with him in the loft, my hand covering his back. Now that he was here, any thought of life without him seemed ridiculous, a mere prelude. Sean had a round head and dark blue eyes. He seemed always on the verge of telling you some joke, a knee-slapper, if only he had the words! His head bobbed eagerly, drool trickled down his chin, his hands circled through the air as if driving a car. He had John's ears and Rhea's nose, John's chin and Rhea's hands, but if I stared at him long enough I saw something of my own expression in his eyes—that dazed, feigned innocence—and a miniature version of Seth's wrinkled forehead.

Life settled, after all, to basics—eating breakfast, tending water lines, digging potatoes out of the ground. Seth and I kept ourselves to our bed, John and Rhea to theirs, and any flare-ups of residual passion were stifled by a glance. Rhea was in charge of this, the only true adult among a gaggle of adolescents. She orchestrated our guilt and grabbed for the baby when he tumbled out of the loft.

She missed. Sean plummeted to the wood floor and Rhea screamed, lunging forward to catch him, a second too late. She told me later that Sean didn't cry at first—he looked stunned and almost smiled—but then he opened his mouth and began a savage wail that did not stop for two hours. Their car screeched by my house in reverse, and all I saw was Sean's wide-open pink mouth, the gums incandescent, and just as John shifted into forward gear I ran closer and pressed my hands on the car window. I saw the lump growing up from Sean's head, and Rhea's breast, mottled and swollen, butting against his cheek. Rhea looked up with a face that dissolved in panic, and I backed off as they swerved onto the road.

They got to the hospital in Ukiah in record time, fifteen minutes on mountain roads that normally take thirty-five, and the doctor said Sean would be fine, the bump looked more awful than it was, there was no permanent damage, and John waited while Rhea pumped the doctor for answers—would Sean be dizzy? would he sleep through the night? should they wake him?—and by that time, Seth and I had shown up and consoled John in the waiting room. Seth rubbed his hand on my shoulder, and I cradled John's head against my chest, and finally Rhea appeared, carrying Sean, and we swarmed around them, Rhea surrendering the baby to me though he still wailed, though his gums still glistened that awful neon pink. John and Seth wrapped their arms around Rhea, and she leaned into each of them in turn, then took the baby from me and brushed her lips against my cheek. Her hair, normally up in a smooth bun, straggled in pieces around her face, and I patted these back behind her ears.

The doctor said Sean would be fine, but Rhea fretted about the falling dreams he might have from then on, as a child and as a man, the terror in the night, the wrench from sleep. She touched the baby's face as he slept, and she worried that he might never be able to love. He might lie with a woman, enraptured, and rise on his elbows to gaze into her face, then reel with a sense of falling, a pain searing through his head. Would he pull away and lie sobbing on the bed, unable to explain? It would sound absurd: *You see, I fell out of the loft when I was three months old....* The women might smile patiently, stroking his back, cooing assurances, but they would leave, one after another; eventually he would just stop trying, and he would hate his mother, she knew it.

I made scrambled eggs while Rhea smoked a cigarette, and John and Seth talked in solemn tones out on the back porch, but they returned looking mischievous; it was late summer and still early morning; out the kitchen windows the rhododendron dripped with dew, and large white buds hovered on the verge of opening. I pointed these out to Rhea and she nodded, her face luminous, and I became awkward then and nearly burned her arm as I scraped the eggs onto her plate. Sean woke while Rhea ate, and I gathered him on the couch, held him against my breast. He rooted there for a time, his nose against my flesh, his fingers drumming. His forehead was damp, and he closed his eyes as he mewed against my skin.

John and Rhea built a railing on the loft, tight-slatted, of birch the color of buttermilk. Seth and I helped, handing up nails, drills, lemonade. I found the process ironically profound—fencing in the site of our historic abandon. Rhea worked grimly, her mouth set in one hard line, but John giggled and pretended to lose his balance, arms windmilling, back arching. *This isn't a game,* Rhea said, invisible in the rafters.

A week later, Seth moved back to Garberville, almost sheepish in his flight. I leaned on the hood of the packed Falcon, mindful of the way the sun lingered on my face. Sean dozed in a sling across my stomach, drooling a quarter-sized spot on my shirt.

Well, I said. Seth had shaved off his beard; his face looked newly hatched. When he bent to kiss me, I smelled eucalyptus and mint so sharp I caught my breath. His cheek against mine was soft and forgiving, a part of him I'd never touched before and now it was gone. He kissed me on the lips, then folded himself around Sean and sobbed. He beeped the horn three times as he backed out to the road. I lifted Sean's hand. We waved.

John moved out of Rhea's place, to a round house balanced on stilts. He wrote music far into the night; sometimes I walked through the woods and saw his candle through the kitchen window. He wrote a song for me, a ballad about rivers swollen beyond their banks. Sean slept fitfully in his bassinet.

The season turned cold overnight, and in the morning frost covered the woodpiles. My house echoed with absence; the walls groaned, and my breath slipped out in a wheeze. I lay in bed a long time, staring at nothing. My fire was hard-starting and flickered uselessly at the logs. I heard Rhea chopping kindling up the road, and I wandered that way, my thighs numb against the inside of my jeans. Rhea stood up the hill, her back to me, the axe swinging high in the air, but the chop-block was empty of wood. She whacked the bare stump again and again. When I reached her she was crying, and I wheedled the ax from her grip. The handle was slick with heat.

She cupped her hands to her face. I stroked her hair, too lightly, but she stopped crying, her body little by little returning to normal, returning to beauty, to the grace she couldn't help. I averted my gaze and stared at her fingers, the tiny knuckles, the half-moon nails even now so perfectly clean. The sight of them filled me with a longing so strong I forgot the cold. *Do you want to come in?* she asked. *Yes,* I said. *Please.*

A year later, Sean fell off the footbridge onto a rocky embankment, but he came up smiling, clutching wildflowers in his fist. A month after that, he fell off the washing machine, breaking a front tooth and spattering his mother and me with blood. After the hospital, Rhea clutched Sean while I fluttered nearby, ineffective, wiping tears and mucus from their cheeks. She rocked the baby, and I made scrambled eggs, then held Sean close to my breast while she ate. Rhea gazed at us both, stroking the baby's feet. *My God,* she whispered, her skin so close to mine it sparked, *how will this child ever survive, how will he learn to love?*

Split

"I could split my heart on the anvil
and put her inside. . . ."
   —Anne Carson
    "Aria of Brittle Failure Theory"

MY HEART, THESE DAYS, IS MUCH TOO DENSE to break. It would require a difficult configuration of tools—mallet, wedge, hatchet, and maul—to make this kind of severance possible. It's tough as those deep knots in the cords of cherry at Orr Hot Springs, those fall days I spent splitting wood outside my cabin, my hands never warm, even under the gloves, even under the heat of the axe. Though I split wood four autumns in that valley, I never felt at ease with the upswing, even more awkward on the downward blow, only every so often getting the clean *thwack* that splits a log in two. More often the steel wedged inside the cleft, and I had to maneuver backward in an awkward little dance—the log hanging off the tip of the axe, me lifting to bang it down again on the stump, then stumbling forward, stumbling back, part struggle, part acquiescence, until the log fell away of its own accord, still intact.

I always felt Seth's eyes on me, even from far away, always felt his not-so-cool appraisal of my stance, my swing. That's why I often longed for a winter heated by nothing but pine: airy wood that yielded so easily under the blade. But such fuel burned too hot, too fast, good only for the quick start of a fire; for the slow burn, the long haul, you need wood that's dense, solid, compact. You need wood that's grown a long time, layer upon layer beneath the bark. They call it heartwood, this core that takes the flame inside and turns it to heat.

When I look at pictures of myself from that time, I'm surprised to find myself smiling so hard, so broadly, my crocheted cap tilted on my head at such a jaunty angle. Surprised this young woman seems so cheerful everywhere she goes: there she is in the garden, shovel in hand, wading through compost up to the knees; at the cistern, with full buckets of water, swinging with one hand off the ladder; on the porch, stacking the wood in geometric cords as if by magic. In all these pictures I seem competent and equanimous; I seem to know what I'm doing, and to like it, but in reality I always bumbled from one task to the next, my face smudged with soot, my shoulders bruised, long splinters speared deep into my palms.

I was the woman men loved to instruct. They'd watch me, bemused, for just as long as it took for all my faults to reveal themselves. Their gazes traveled over my body, past the layers of flannel and wool, past the damp undershirt and to the girl-flesh that lay beneath, my nipples breathtakingly hard, my breath fluttering inside my chest. I wish I'd known, then, the difference between love and valuation, knew enough to take the axe firmly in hand and aim not for the wood but for the block on which it rests, to slice through the log as if knots were only a matter of perspective. But the men got to me first. They walked over, their legs so assured inside their jeans; they put a hand on my shoulder and turned me just a bit with the slightest touch. *Here, honey,* they said, their voices a gentle mutter to the heart, *here's how it's done.* They stood behind me and gripped the axe in both our hands; they lifted it high above our heads—the steel a blur of motion, of light—and showed me the proper way to split.

Artifacts

Angel

Once, in Sonoma, I bought an angel suspended from a twig. Her head is a polished knob of wood the size of my thumb; her hair, a mass of curly white thread. Her body's a thin shave of wood the color of cream. She's surrounded by strings of gold stars, and in her arms more stars cluster, overflowing. I know this mobile's supposed to dangle over a child's crib, dispensing blessing, but I have no child. So it hovers in a corner of my bedroom, and I watch from my bed, late at night: the twisting stars, the oblivious angel.

I saw it in a toy store on Main Street, while walking with Sean. We glanced sidelong at each other as we loitered until his father got off work. I wanted to hold his hand, but I didn't dare; he was eight years old, a man already, and as we browsed the store windows we grunted to each other in low, indecipherable voices. At the toy store Sean wanted to buy a present for his mother and, with relief, we went our separate ways. He looked at clay earrings and stuffed monkeys; I touched this angel with my fingertip, tracing the black-marker crescents of her eyes, the red dot of her mouth.

As the angel drifted in her limited circle, I thought about Sean's birth, in the round shack at Orr Hot Springs, his head crowning, the turned shoulders, the body rollicking onto the bloody sheet. I remembered holding him twenty minutes later, in the rocking chair by the window as the morning ascended outside the glass. He still smelled of the womb; he tapped his white, wrinkled fingers against his lower lip, like an old man reminiscing. His gaze seemed all peripheral, and as I stared at him I said words I've never said before or since.

Of course Sean's forgotten, but I know he remembers *something*. As a toddler he sometimes looked at me oddly and babbled about our "special place," asked me to take him there. I walked with him down to the bend in the river and threw stones into the water, kneeling with him in the wild grass.

I went back to the store later, alone, and bought the angel for five dollars. The saleslady asked if it was a present, if I would like it wrapped, and I said, oh yes, that would be nice. It attracts whatever light seeps into the bedroom, fragments light into octagonal bits of stars. The angel's eyes are always closed; her mouth forever open in a red "Oh," which I take to mean singing, but could just as easily be surprise, admonition, a yawn.

Shell

A fragment of a snail shell, bleached white, the whorl in the middle a bluish brown that sprouts to a point like a diminutive nipple. I found it on Whidbey Island, on a cold February afternoon. I had my own cottage in the woods, and in the mornings I sat in the window seat and wrote letters to my friends about the progress of the forced hyacinth I had brought with me from Seattle: *Its folded body still so green...I feel like that bulb, just now opening, but perhaps before my time....* I wrote to them about growing older, about my fear of being alone and childless as I aged.

I usually grew discouraged in the afternoons, when the light no longer looked so promising through the pines, and so I got on my bicycle and pedaled for seven or eight miles along the coastal road, churning up hills, past gardens with stuffed owls to keep away the starlings. Or sometimes I just rode a mile to Useless Bay, and walked there at low tide, watching the sanderlings scuttle out of my path.

The shell was buried in the sand, the same color as the sand, camouflaged. I unearthed it and put it on my windowsill, gazed at it till it hypnotized me. Sometimes it became an eye, staring back, asking me to go deeper, to follow that spiral path into the center. Sometimes it disappeared in the dome light of afternoon. Other shells lay scattered on the path outside my cottage door, disintegrating under my feet, scattering into mosaic. Intertwined with the broken bodies lay feathers from the legs of an owl, dried needles of fir, cedar cones, footprints of invisible deer.

Crystal

In the garden of my house at Orr Hot Springs I dug up a round crystal while trying to dig under the compost. I struck it with the edge of my spade, picked it out of the dirt, brought it inside, and washed it at the kitchen sink. I strung it with a piece of mint-green dental floss, hung it in the loft window. Seth came upstairs as I touched it, as it threw truncated rainbows across the sun-yellow ceiling. *Look what I found,* I said, and he said, *Lovely,* then kissed me behind the ears, down my neck to the place where the change begins, where the head becomes the body, and the body knows nothing of its own bounds. I lay back with him—our love already disintegrating, turning to shards dangerous and elusive as glass. But he traced the scar below my belly button, his fingers inexplicably kind, forgiving. My crystal knocked against the window, twisted on its string, transformed whatever light happened to fall upon our skin.

Dead People's Things

My grandfather's silverware, adorned with roses, the initial "M" engraved in the handle of each utensil. My grandmother's linen handkerchiefs, monogrammed with the same "M," yellowed around the edges. Books from people I never knew, bought at bookstores with dusty shelves and dim lights, the inscriptions on the flyleaves sheared of any luster, sad now in the wrong hands. A wedding photograph of my grandmother and grandfather, my grandmother's hands covered in flowers, her eyes focused on a place that does not include me.

Empty Vessels

A glazed bowl from Mendocino, swirled in pastels of blue and pink; a green-striped pitcher from Portugal; a blue vase from Italy, the glass pale and veined with ivy; a reed and willow basket from Montana, braids of acorns dangling from the handle. I like the fact of their emptiness; not only the clean lines of the vessels themselves, sharp against their backdrops, but the empty space they shape and contain. I'm tempted to leave these vessels empty forever, to forgo the cut flowers, the coins, the fruit.

My Zen teacher told me "emptiness is form and form is emptiness," a phrase I repeated but never understood until now, as I lie on my rug in my new apartment and gaze at these forms which keep changing under my eye. One moment they are clearly containers; the next moment they are contained by what encircles them. I've often thought of my body as empty, in a negative way: I've seen the cup of my pelvis as a dark, vaguely malevolent, void. But now I start to sense the lovely shape of these bones as a container for the body that surrounds them.

Two people I know died in their sleep this week. As I think about them, their empty bodies float in my mind—sometimes light, unfettered; sometimes heavy and inert as lead. Both died of heart failure: a forty-nine-year-old woman and a nineteen-year-old girl. And, as I surround myself with empty vessels, I become aware of my own heartbeat, the shallow labor of my lungs against my ribs. *Form is emptiness, emptiness form,* I repeat to myself, and with that hymn my body starts to hum, to be filled.

Infant Ward

THIS CHILD IS NOT MY OWN, but still the words of possession slip from me: *my baby girl, my sweet baby.* I've never seen her before this minute, but I think I know what she needs: the lights at her hospital bedside dimmed, her loose arms girdled securely against her chest. This patient has no name except "Girl _____," a family surname typed on the identification card at the end of her crib. She's too young, too early, to have a name like Betty, or Jennifer, or Anastasia. She surprised everyone, caught her parents without a crib or a car seat, without the casseroles in the freezer, without the stamina. I pat her back, I shade her eyes, I clutch both her hands in my palm, strong against her sternum. She relaxes and makes a sound—not a laugh or a sob, but something in between—a sigh moist with resignation.

It's a moment of simple communication, common here on the infant ward at Children's Hospital. I gurgle back to her and so we converse, our rudimentary voices vibrating the cord that governs reflex. Conflict resolution is reduced to this: she sticks out her tongue;

I stick out mine. She blinks; I blink. She makes a gurgled moan, and so do I. She cries, and my voice veers up in commiseration: *Yes, I know, everything's going to be all right.*

Though, of course, I know no such thing. I know nothing about her except her immediate physical needs and desires. I don't know which organs are failing, or if there are gaps that weaken her heart, or where her parents might be. I'm just a volunteer; every Wednesday I put on a blue jacket with my name tag, then I hold babies for three hours. *I'm just a volunteer,* I say when a parent mistakenly asks me about medications, or when a doctor arrives to pass his flashlight across a baby's face. That "just" modifies me; I become a presence inconspicuous yet necessary as a ceiling tile, or a light.

I know nothing, and in lieu of knowledge I cultivate instinct. I slip through the halls, almost invisible, drawn by a baby's cry anywhere on the floor. I snap on the latex gloves. I bend and thread my arms through a tangle of i.v. lines and lift the child away from her crib. I back myself into a rocking chair, by now an expert at holding the array of tubing aloft, hardly noticing anymore the bandages, the bruises, the cuts. The baby might promptly fall asleep, but I go on rocking and rocking. I can't put her down, not yet. I know she feels me rocking even in her sleep. I hope she drifts into a dream of comfort and love without surcease. Her breath—sour and bitter—becomes my breath, her stuttering heart my own.

Or she might stay awake, gazing at me and wondering. I rock "Girl _____" for two hours. The motion reminds me of the davening of Jewish men at the front of the synagogue: the repeated half-bow to an unseen presence, the bodily gesture of prayer. The baby blinks slowly, her fingers tug at the oxygen tube in her nose, her pupils expand just slightly when they alight on my face. Three different i.v. bags dispense liquids drop by drop. The tubes converge into a single needle piercing the back of her hand, held rigid by a padded splint. A nurse beckons to me, so I lift the child back into her crib, place her on her side, and tuck a rolled blanket against her back. I watch her a few seconds more, my chest already cold with her absence. I know, if she's lucky, we'll never see each other again.

The nurse asks me to help pacify a distressed preemie, and I slip my hands through the gloves in the incubator and stroke a stomach the size of a newborn kitten's. He's crying, but I barely hear him through the plastic walls, and soon he settles down: his arms lie open at his side, his mouth shapes itself to an imaginary breast.

Around me, the ward projects an aura of stability—no emergencies here, no alarm. One floor above us lies Intensive Care: many of the babies descend from that plane, returned from the brink, their parents exhausted and pale. One floor below is the emergency room: many of the babies ascend from there, successfully returned from seizures, choking, concussion. Sandwiched between the floors of panic lies this base of equilibrium, with its multiple i.v. stands, chairs rocking, babies sleeping, every breath monitored, every pulse— many of the patients so small they're only a swell of blankets in the middle of these vast hospital cribs. We're surrounded by the mesh of protocol: nurses slip from task to task, swaddling a baby in an instant, stripping paper off thermometers, writing every observation in their charts—these actions merge into one, and they lull me into feeling that all is business as usual, nothing could really go wrong.

But in one of the isolation rooms a child is screaming: a little girl, two days old, born with no anus. "She poops out the same hole as she pees," the nurse cheerfully tells me, in case I need to change her. I sit in the rocking chair, holding the newborn as she grimaces. I can't help it, I become acutely conscious of my own body: my colon, my vagina, my rectum; I imagine how easy it would be for something to go wrong, for the parts not to match up completely. One small error, and a lifetime of pain, discomfort, complication. Maybe not even that. Maybe not a lifetime.

Sleeper couches fold out next to each crib, and often the floor space surrounding them is cluttered with overnight bags, magazines, bags of snacks. In these cribs, Polaroid photos of Mom and Dad hang at eye level, crayon drawings by siblings chirp *I love you!*, and colorful handmade blankets are tucked into corners.

When no parents stand at these bedsides, I wonder where they are. I wonder where I would be if my baby were in a hospital crib, attached to a monitor to make sure she was alive. If my baby were in the hospital for three months, would I have the stamina to sleep in one of these white leatherette chairs every night? Would I walk outside under the blossoming cherry trees that line the driveway of Children's Hospital? Would I keep walking, down to Lake Washington, and on and on, gulping the fresh air, trying not to scream? I don't know. I want to believe I would be at the bedside every minute, holding my child against my belly. But, yesterday I had a splitting headache, and I wanted nothing more than to put down the fussing baby at my shoulder. I wanted nothing more than to be unburdened beneath the cherry trees.

Most often the cribs I approach are steely blank, the baby wearing a hospital issue T-shirt, the only decoration on the crib an identification card and a densely scribbled chart. No balloons, no photos, no drawings—only plain, flannel blankets from the hospital shelves. This naked bed usually signals that the child has been abandoned, left to the care of the hospital or the systems that stand in place for such infants. The parents cannot be found, or refuse to come, or are under arrest.

Today I walk by an isolation room where the I.D. card reads: "Doe, Jane." Beneath this card, a green slip of paper asks the parents or guardians of this child to come to Admitting and fill out the requisite paperwork. I know this means the parents have disappeared. The shades are drawn; the door, closed. I hover a moment but hear no cry, nothing to demand my presence, so I move on, my hands pushed deep into the square pockets of my blue jacket.

In the next room there is a baby girl born too early, at thirty weeks, to a teen-ager who received no prenatal care. The baby's bones were so brittle most of them fractured during delivery; now she's almost blind, her lungs are malformed, her hearing damaged. But, two months out of the womb, she seems determined to live: she sucks on her bottle voraciously, tugging the nipple into her mouth, her eyes popping. The mother has not visited for three weeks, a student nurse tells me, and so I automatically hold the baby closer, whisper in her ear, as if she needs it more than the others, as if these few hours could somehow make up for a lifetime's worth of neglect.

When I get home I tell my boyfriend about this child, about her medical problems and the absent mother. He responds: "Why didn't the mother just get an abortion?" And since he has spoken my hidden thoughts, the ones I've tried to suppress all afternoon, I become angry and leave the dinner table. I go out on the front steps and cry. When he comes out to apologize, I say: *That baby is not an abstract concept anymore.*

After my three months on this floor, the question of abortion has become more troubling to me, has sharpened into the one essential question: when did the few, divided cells inside a teen-aged girl become that baby whose weight I still felt in my arms? Certainly the girl might have been better off choosing abortion; perhaps her child is destined for nothing but a life of trouble and pain. But is there really some threshold between nonhuman and human that is crossed at three months, four months, or six? Does a fetus become human only when it looks like a person, with hands and fingers and hair? How do I explain the grief I still feel at my own miscarriages? The embryos were only four weeks old, but I still have the nagging sense that something—something human—has been irretrievably lost.

I have no answers, but I have too much time to question such things while I rock back and forth, these babies breathing rapidly in my arms. Some of them look as though they're still in the womb, they're that wrinkled and tenuous. I pat my hand rhythmically between their shoulder blades. I mimic an intrauterine heartbeat, giving the babies one overriding stimulus around which to organize chaos.

Sometimes they stop breathing a moment, suspended, and I panic. I nudge them a little, and their breath starts up, normal, smelling of milk. Their chapped lips twitch up into the reflex of a smile.

To volunteer, they say, is to be aligned with the fullness of your own volition. The term "volunteer" stems from the obsolete word "voluty" which means "that which one wishes or desires." You do this work because it comes from you naturally; if that impulse falters, you may stop, no questions asked. The volunteer tomatoes in my garden grow without any prompting from me; they arrive out of nowhere, and the volunteers are the hardiest ones, sticking it out long past the others have withered from drought or flood or disease.

We glance sideways at each other, us volunteers. We see the blue jackets out the corners of our eyes and nod. We come for different reasons, I know, though the motives all reduce to two or three identical lines on the application forms: *I want to give something back to the community. I love kids. I'm interested in being a doctor.* Hovering behind these lines are the other reasons: *I'm lonely. I'm childless. I want to feel as if I matter. I want to be missed when I'm gone.*

I don't know if I'm missed when I'm gone. I get in my car and remove the blue jacket, the name tag. My hands smell like baby, or of the soap at the ward sink, a vaguely nauseating combination of hospital and the insides of latex gloves lined with talc. My left arm will be sore for a day; I'll live the rest of the week mostly inside my office, writing, or going to the health club, riding my bicycle through the city streets to the bay. Then comes Tuesday. My schedule takes on a pleasing and necessary weight. "Tomorrow I'm at the hospital," I say to no one in particular, marking it again on the calendar.

Yesterday I held a baby who'd been beaten into a coma. I held her for my entire shift, her body unnaturally rigid, her cry like a cat's meow. Her nerves could still respond to pain, the nurse told me, but otherwise her brain was absent, her pupils fixed. She was six months old. "Doesn't look like she'll come out of it," the nurse said. She touched the baby's head gently, then left me alone with her. This girl seemed most comfortable nestled tightly against my side, while I remained motionless; any movement startled her reflexes and made her cry. Once, she sucked her pacifier for twenty minutes, this instinct bypassing the dead circuits in her brain. I memorized her eyelashes—deep black and impossibly long, curling against the ridge of her cheek.

I couldn't help but imagine the scene—the moment the large hand struck the soft spot at her temple, the impact, the crack of bone. I held her in the crook of my arm; I became rigid, like her, stiff as a catatonic. Hours later, when the nurses and I finally wedged the girl upright in bed, I saw her face full-on for the first time. She was awake: one eye wide open, the other halfway closed. Her pupils blank. Her tongue resting mute inside her mouth.

When I left the hospital, I sat in my car and cried from exhaustion and fury. I drove home, my hands white against the steering wheel. I made dinner. I went to a movie. My boyfriend said: "Perhaps you will be a blip on her memory, a second of comfort." Perhaps. "Do you know how," he said, "when you're sick, and what you remember from those days is the hour a cool breeze came through the curtains, cooling you? That moment of relief?"

More likely I'll be nothing, or only a part of the continuum of pain. All that night I felt this baby's weight on my arm. I remembered stroking her knee, her calf, her toes already stiff, as if in rigor mortis. I remembered that one eye, open wide, but focused on nothing. I could not reach her. While I stroked her, I tried to explain: *This is what touch can mean.*

I am there only once a week. I hold usually one baby, maybe two, sometimes three. How do these nurses bear it, the doctors? I want to ask them, but they're too busy. The babies keep coming, arriving from Intensive Care, from the emergency room. Like sponges, the babies absorb all a family's frustration, an entire community's pain. They emerge, tactile evidence of abstract phenomena: here is the mottled face of poverty, there the body of abuse. Here are the hands of racism, inequity, and impotence— bruised from the repeated probe of an i.v.

Today is my last day on the infant ward. I'm moving to Salt Lake City, and I know I'm going to miss these children more than I can say. The nurse, whose name I've never learned, has asked me to hold a little girl two months old, tiny as a newborn. This baby has a deep, phlegmy cough, so I need to wear a gown, gloves, and a full facial mask to feed her the bottle. She stares at me, astonished, grinning so much the nipple keeps popping from between her lips. The world to her is all eyes, looming above pink paper masks, and I can sense her trying to strip these masks away with the force of her gaze. She wears a hospital issue T-shirt, and socks that slither up her calves like leg warmers. No books, balloons, or drawings decorate her room. I see no name on her chart.

Who are you? I ask her, smiling under my mask. The nipple slides from her mouth. Her eyes are so bright I can hardly bear to look at them. They will burn me, I think, excavate all my fear and desire. But I lean a little closer to hear what she might say. Her arms windmill around her head—pointing out the window to the cherry trees, to the other babies, to the nurses, and back to me. She keeps her gaze steady on my face. *Who are you?* she asks.

Who am I? I am a woman holding a baby not my own. I take her weight, light as it is, and hold her the way mothers will always hold infants: close to the breast, the heart.

PART THREE

A Brief History of Sex

"Why haven't I
thought of it before?
This body,
remembering yours,
is the keepsake you left."
—Izumi Shikibu

I.

A Japanese courtesan waits in her room: the walls, so thin, translucent, cannot contain her desire. It is morning in the eleventh century, a morning damp with dew in the long grasses. Her body? Well, her body smells faintly of almonds and musk. This body, so thin, translucent, cannot contain her desire, or memory: they drift as fog somewhere above the lattice, the garden, the stream. She waits for the letter her lover will send by messenger, any moment now, perhaps wrapped in a lotus petal, or tied with bamboo to a branch of flowering cherry. Even now his hand (sweet memory) calligraphs the words carefully on rice paper, the same hand that inscribed itself on her skin. She tries to remember a face, but he was so close all night, too close to see; he deliquesces into the mien of the lovers before him, the lovers to come. She sighs. She looks to the wooden pillow, the tousled bed, then outside to the silk threads veiling the chrysanthemums, the jeweled net of the forsythia. She waits. She is a lady-in-waiting. His letter could be a question. Might ask: "My love, the lilies—how many may bloom in a single pond?"

II.

How many have come before me, my love? They ask me in cars, in cafés, in bed. I ask them at breakfast, at dinner, at tea. It's only a matter of time: that question will be asked, if only silently, if only by an unguarded glance. "How many?" he asks, coyly, a little shy, as if this question were all in fun, not serious, means nothing at all. "How many have you *known?*" He may want only an approximate number, rounded off to the nearest zero; or he may want names and dates and positions and if you really loved them and how could you know?

You must analyze the question carefully, because a correct answer does exist, in the air between you. If you get it wrong, this test, the results could be disastrous. You have to think a moment. A pause to go back over the tapes in your head, rewinding and stopping. You might need clarification: what counts and what doesn't? Duration? Penetration? Foreplay?

Sometimes I know the right answer, and say it aloud, casually, unafraid, with a modest downturn of the head. But sometimes it's a trick. They don't really want these witnesses in your bed: perched on the pillows, the wainscoting, the drawers. You have to lie a little, fudge the facts, reveal them one at a time, the way you do the scars on your body, each scar a story, each mark not an accretion but the site of an excavation, a taking away.

I count them like coins, finger them like pearls sewn on a collar or a sleeve. If I say the names aloud it will be a spell, words that summon and sustain. Let's see: there was Mark and Dan and Jeff, Carolyn and Rhea, Karl and Pat and John (am I getting close, is this what you want?), the guy with no name, and Keith and Joel (I know I'm forgetting someone, or something...). They begin to pile up on the stairs behind me, each of them shearing a bit of my skin. My own name must be lost in their litanies, too, as they lie with their wives and their husbands and lovers, morning fast upon them as they speak. And there I go, so quickly, two syllables at least, a pause.

III.

Now Adam knew Eve his wife....

I know you, he says. I know everything about you. He takes her once again into his arms, presses her to the wound in his side; the birds of paradise look on, and the snake. Leaves rustle in the Tree of Life, a large ginkgo perhaps, tree of memory, with leaves the color and shape of silk fans. The four rivers flow in a helix around them, babbling among pebbles of onyx and gold. ... *and they become one flesh. And the man and his wife were both naked, and were not ashamed.* She looks into his eyes; he looks into hers; they are the same person, the same, intersecting in the before-time, before the dalliance with the snake, before the taste of anything but each other, before all the names and the begetting, that furious chain of reproduction. He asks her nothing. No question hangs in the air between them, perfect virgins, unkissed and new, naked in front of God and everyone.

IV.

as if a thousand penitents
kissed an icon
till it thinned
back to bare wood.
            —Jane Hirshfield

I sleep alone in my double bed while others have sex below the eaves, their animal cries more whimpers than pleasure. How many women like me sit at their kitchen tables and cover their faces with their hands, afraid even this will be taken from us finally: our eyes, our imperfect sight. We sleep alone but something musses our hair in the night, strokes us into dishevelment, so in the morning our mirrors give back a person foreign and wild. We are loosened, and it's all I want, in the end, to blow in a breeze and be lovely the few moments it takes for someone to see and pass on. My face at some window, always looking and sometimes, *oh rarely!*, looked upon.

I remember my hand moving to touch a shoulder but not the moment of contact, and it's what I want again, and again: the *almost* of any desire, that impetus to reach.

If anyone asks, tell them my tongue these days is silent as a fish resting in a gravel bed. It stirs sometimes to feed, but then drops heavily to the bottom of the stream. If anyone asks, tell them: hunger is best unsatisfied. If anyone asks, tell them: light is always in the process of arrival. If they ask, tell them I would speak but for the stones that lately settle in my throat. I don't mind, tell them, it was all so gradual, this silencing. It keeps me from mistaking speech for truth. It keeps me from speaking too soon of desire.

I've been kissed but kisses do not linger. The skin's new every seven years, so any love we accumulate is sloughed off with the rest. Even if you gather the peelings, they'll never make good wood again. Think of yourself as heartwood: the core of the tree where the sap no longer runs. Blood's necessary only for that which changes and sheds. Be like the well-loved icon, stripped bare by kisses, more holy for its lack of adornment.

V.

Krishna meets his *gopi* lover Radha in the temple at Khajuraho. Krishna plays his flute, or dances his three-bend dance on the head of a conquered snake. He's a charmer, and Radha knows it; she dances toward him, envy of all the girls, wrapped in her acres of silk. Among the lotus flowers, among the frolicking cows, under a moon that's a mandala, they meet. *I know you*, he says, *I know everything about you.* He asks her nothing. They writhe in stone: she twisted full-length on top of him, her face turned up in a profile of perfect content, mouth swollen for still another kiss. It's his face we see full on, eyes closed, his index finger and thumb not quite joined on her backside in a mudra of peace. He gives her his bad-boy smile. *Oh good one*, she laughs, *oh Krishna.* The circle unclosed means the spirit revealed, and he plants it there, on the peach of her body. She barely feels it there, in her ecstasy. The gods smile in stone, dead and alive, a forgetting and a remembering all at once.

VI.

The scrapbooks, the photo albums, the conversations over wine about movies and food: they only go so far. And so I took off my clothes so they could see me better, and I lay down on the bed (the sofa, the floor) so they could touch me better, and I opened my mouth so they could taste me better. I said the names. I revealed my scars to them, one by one, those carvings in stone, that text in the flesh, and invited them to read, to study, to learn. If they ask, I'll tell them: I want their bodies to scour my own. I want the heat of them to purge me, distill me to nothing but a fragrant smoke.

It's like a riddle: What gives and gives and still takes away? When is addition really subtraction? How many lovers does it take to screw in a lightbulb?

TRUE OR FALSE: A lover is someone who loves.

WORD PROBLEM: If a woman's had 15 lovers, and if each lover loved her for an average of 48 weeks, how much love has this woman accumulated in her lifetime? How much will this love weigh? (Note: use the value and measure of love determined by the current economy.)

VII.

They ask me how many. C'mon, how many? One, two, twelve? The test is given, and I, the good student, the pupil with furrowed brow,

I bend to the task with quiet fortitude and resilience. I sit with this test before me, chewing my pen. All my life I've been told a correct answer joins to every question. The two make reason for the other to exist, just as a lover presupposes the existence of love. A question with no answer? It makes the heart beat uncertainly in the chest. A lover with no love? It makes an ache in the jaw that descends from the open eye.

How many lovers does it take to screw in a lightbulb? None, they make their own light. I bend my head to the test. My pupils widen. The gray circle round my iris darkens, as it does when I'm close to tears. Unknowing does me no good. My pen is poised in the air, ready to write what I know, when I know it. How many lilies bloom in a single pond? How much water will it take to sustain them? What happens when they're no longer beautiful, when no one can see them in the dusk?

It's not the questions I fear, but the pause afterward. That ticking silence, when answers have yet to arrive.

Prologue to a Sad Spring

I'VE PUT A NEW PICTURE ON MY WALL, a photograph bought for me at an Edward Weston exhibit last April. The composition shows a young woman, all in black, posed against a high, white fence. She half turns toward the camera; her right hand lies tentatively across her heart. The shadow of a leafless tree (I imagine it to be a young oak) curves up and over this slight figure. Actually, it does more than curve; the tree arches across the tall fence in a gesture of protection. Almost a bow of respect.

A wide-brimmed hat, trimmed in flowers, overshadows the woman's face, but I can make out the line of her small chin, the pensive set of her mouth. She seems to gaze at some person beyond the camera, someone who moves away quite rapidly, and she can't quite decide whether to follow. It is a moment of suppressed panic. Even in her frame, the woman appears to tremble.

Why do I like this picture so much? I glance at it every day, and every day it puzzles me. What draws me to those dark, shaded eyes?

What holds me transfixed by the movement of gray shadows over the straight white planks, the drape of the black coat, the white hand raised to the breast in a stunned gesture of surprise or healing?

Weston called this photo *Prologue to a Sad Spring*, and I think it's the title that gets to me, rivets me to this vague woman and her fluttering hand. So many questions in that phrase, so much tragedy touched upon. I know April is Eliot's cruel month, and Dickinson "dreaded that first robin so. . . ." Edna St. Vincent Millay growled that "April/Comes like an idiot, babbling and strewing flowers." But I want it to be different; I want spring to redeem us from the weight of other seasons. To be sad in the fall is understandable, even appropriate, given all the reminders of death, the withering garden; to be sad in the winter is the accepted state of affairs. To be sad in the summer is not unthinkable, given the unrelenting and often cheerless sun. But to be sad in the spring is to renounce what the season ostensibly stands for. To be sad in the spring—amid a fever of cherry blossoms, a dusting of lilacs—this hints at a grief that is inconsolable.

And prologue. It is only the beginning. A long, sad spring stretches before her, this woman in the photo I'm so taken with. Perhaps her lover left in the early days of spring, to return to a distant home. Perhaps she realized the strength of their love only in the moment of turning away. And so—the hand to the breast, the quick surprise of pain, the helpless glance backward in hope that he is still there, that someone will be there, that surely she cannot be alone on this cold, colorless April day.

But that is the stuff of foreign novels and old movies. Anna Karenina could be caught in such a pose, as she waits for her tardy lover Vronksy in Vrede's garden. She could pull off the restrained elegance, the striking presence. Bacall waiting for Bogart could drape herself in just such tragic lines. For myself, I've never been lucky enough to be caught against a white backdrop, that moment of pain exposed by a trick of the light, a turn of the head. When I am sad in the spring, there is no tall fence for me to lean against, no young oak to throw an embracing shadow. My sorrow remains common and dull, expressing itself at odd moments and rarely with the dignity the woman in this picture possesses.

When I am sad in the spring, I scrub the windows hard to dispel the grime of winter, then sit with the windows closed to gather the effect of light through the polished panes. I pose on the white couch and watch for the correct slant of sun and shadow across the lake. When the light plays across my face just right, I sit and deliberate on my sadness completely. But no observer is there to frame the moment into significance, and so my unhappiness passes through the world without notice.

When my lover leaves in the early days of spring, when I realize something important has slipped away again, you will not find a photo of me with chin upraised, a hand laid calmly over the heart, illuminated. Instead I am hidden in a back room, in a heap on the bed, disheveled, talking myself into tears and wondering, like all fools before me, if I will ever be loved again. The ache pools in the palms of my hands, the bottoms of my feet. My hand may fly to my heart, but it does not stay there long; my suffering has no art to it.

Perhaps it would if I lived in soft-focus black and white, if I could strip away the hard grainy details of my life and return to vague, romantic impressions. Like this woman and her tree. Edward Weston once wrote that "black-and-white photography has, at the start, an advantage over color in that it is already a step removed from a factual rendition of the scene." Perhaps this woman is really dressed all in red, and the fence behind her painted a bright blue.

The shadows would not be so alluring, then; I don't think I would care quite so much. As it is, I find the tree's shadow to be the most intriguing part of the picture. It has the most mystery to it, and the most promise. With the strong curve of the trunk, the sinuous movement of the limbs overhead, the tree forms a vigilant presence, a sentinel. The oak dominates the scene, carries all the light, draws the eye to this woman, who, in her preoccupation, keeps looking the opposite way.

The Date

When I return naked to the stone porch,
there is no one to see me glistening.

—Linda Gregg

A MAN I LIKE IS COMING FOR DINNER TONIGHT. This means I sleep very little, and I wake up in the half-light of dawn, disoriented, wondering where I am. I look at my naked body stretched diagonally across the bed; I look at the untouched breasts, the white belly, and I wonder. I don't know if this man will ever touch me, but I wonder.

I get up, and I make coffee. While I wait for the water to boil I vaguely study the pictures and poems and quotes held in place by magnets on my refrigerator. I haven't really looked at these things in a long time, my gaze usually blinking out as I reach for the refrigerator door. This morning I try to look at these objects clearly, objectively, as if I were a stranger, trying to figure what this man will think of them and so, by extension, what he will make of me.

He'll see pictures of my three nieces, my nephew, my godson. He'll see my six women friends hiking in a slot canyon of the San Rafael swell, straddling the narrow gap with their strong thighs, their muscular arms. He'll see the astrological forecast for Pisces ("There's never been a better moment to turn your paranoia into *pronoia*," it insists), and the Richard Campbell quote which tells me if I'm to live like a hero I must be ready at any moment, "there is no other way." He'll see Rumi: "Let the Beauty we love be what we do. There are hundreds of ways to kneel and kiss the ground." He'll see me kayaking with my friend Kathy in the San Juan Islands, and then, if his gaze moves in a clockwise direction, he'll see me sitting with my parents inside the Oasis Cafe in Salt Lake City. He'll glance at me standing on the estate of Edna St. Vincent Millay, my arms around my fellow artist colonists, grinning as if I were genuinely happy.

Who is this person on my refrigerator door? Every morning, these bits and pixels try to coalesce into a coherent image, a picture for me to navigate by as I move solitary through my morning routine of coffee, juice, cereal, a few moments of blank rumination out the stained-glass kitchen window. I suppose we put these things on our refrigerators as subliminal reminders of self, to fortify those parts of the self most necessary to get us through a day. But I've seen these fragments so often they've come to mean nothing to me; I barely see them, and I know this collage exists only for others, a constructed persona for the few people who make it this far into my house, my kitchen, my life. *Look*, it says, *look how athletic/spiritual/creative/loved I am.* And my impulse, though I stifle it, is to rearrange all these items: delete some, add others, in order to create a picture I think this man will like.

But how could I know? How would I keep from making a

mistake? Besides, I tell myself, a mature woman would never perform such a silly and demeaning act. So I turn away from the fridge, leave things the way they are. I drink my coffee and gaze out the window. It's February, and the elm trees are bare, the grass brown under patches of snow. Tomorrow is Valentine's Day, a fact I've been avoiding. I think about the blue tulips I planted in the fall, still hunkered underground, and the thought of them in the darkness, their pale shoots nudging the hard-packed soil, makes me a little afraid.

I'm thirty-eight years old, and I've been alone for almost three years now, have dated no one since leaving my last boyfriend, who is now marrying someone else in California. Sometimes I like to be alone; I come into my bedroom, pleased by the polish of light through the half-closed venetian blinds. I lie on my bed at odd hours of the day with a small lavender pillow over my eyes, like the old woman I think I'm becoming. At times like these, the light in my bedroom seems a human thing, kind and forgiving, and my solitude a position to be envied, guarded even if it means I will remain unpartnered for life.

But this feeling of "unpartneredness" can set me adrift in a way that frightens me. I gaze into my bedroom and see no light, smell no lavender. Instead, the empty room throbs like a reproach—dark, unyielding. I can't move beyond the threshold; I stand there, paralyzed, panic gnawing beneath my skin. I try to breathe deeply, try to remember the smiling self on my refrigerator door, but that person seems all surface, a lie rehearsed so many times it bears faint semblance to truth. I cry as if every love I've known has been false somehow, a trick.

At these times I want only to be part of the coupled universe, attached to some cornice that might solidify my presence in a world which too often renders me invisible. In my parents' house an entire wall is devoted to formal family photographs, and the family groupings fall into neat, symmetrical lines: my older brother, his wife and two children flanking one side of my parents; my younger brother, his wife and two children balance out the other. When I lived with my boyfriend Keith for five years, my parents insisted we take a portrait as well, and we did: me in a green T-shirt and multicolored beads, Keith in jeans and a denim shirt, standing with our arms entwined. So for a while, my photo, and my life, fit neatly into the familial constellation.

Keith and I split up, but the photo remained on the wall a year longer, staring down at me when I came to visit for Hanukkah. "You have to take that down," I finally told them, and they nodded sadly, said "we know." Now a portrait of myself, alone, hangs in its place—a nice photograph, flattering, but it still looks out of line amid the growing and changing families that surround it. Whenever I visit, my young nephew asks me, "Why aren't you married?" and gazes at me with a mixture of wonder and alarm.

A man I like is coming to dinner, and so I get out all my cookbooks and choose and discard recipes as if trying on dresses. I want something savory yet subtle, not too messy, not too garlicky, just in case we kiss. I don't know if we'll kiss, but just in case. I don't know much about this man at all. I know he has two young daughters, an ex-wife; he writes poetry, and teaches a hundred high school students every day. I don't know how old he is, but I suspect he's younger than I am, and so I need to be careful not to reveal too much too fast.

It will be our third date, this dinner. From what I've heard, the third date's either the charm or the poison. I have a friend who in the last five years has never "gotten past the third date." She calls me at 10:30 on a Friday night. "Third date syndrome," she sighs.

She describes the sheepish look on her date's face as she returns to the table after a trip to the Ladies' room. She tells me about the "Let's just be friends speech" that by now she has memorized: "You're great. I enjoy your company, but a) I don't have a lot of time right now, b) I'm not looking for a relationship, c) I'm going to be out of town a lot in the next couple of months." My friend sighs and tells me: "I just wish one of them would come right out and say, 'Look, I don't really like you. Let's just forget it.' It would be a relief."

I listen to her stories with a morbid fascination, the way I might listen to a friend's travel adventures: the wrong turn into the Men's bathroom in a bus station in Turkey, the fish heads staring out at you from a plate of stew in Italy. I listen to her stories with both wonder and relief, as if she is traveling in some dangerous land to which I've, thankfully, been denied a visa.

But then we hang up and I turn back to my empty house, the bed whose wide expanse looks accusatory in my bedside light, the pile of books that has grown lopsided and dangerous. I stare at my fish, a fighting fish named Betty, who flares his gills at me and swims in vicious circles around his plastic hexagon, whips his iridescent body back and forth. My friend Connie tells me this behavior indicates love, that my fish is expressing his masculinity so I might want to mate with him. I take this explanation as a compliment.

A man I like is coming to dinner, which means I need to do the laundry and wash the sheets, just in case. I don't know how long it's been since I washed the sheets. There's been no need to keep track. It's just me here after all, and I'm always clean when I go to bed, fresh from the bath; nothing happens in that bed to soil it. When I lived with Seth, or Keith, I washed the sheets every week, but then I had someone in the laundromat to help me fold them when they were dry.

As I dangle the dry sheets over the Laundromat's metal table, I realize that I've never really dated before. I've always been transparent: approach me and you see inside. Touch me and I will open, like a door made of rice paper, light and careless. It's difficult to remember the beginnings of things; was there always this dithering back and forth, this wondering, this not-knowing? On my first date with my first boyfriend, Kevin, we took LSD and sat in a tree for five hours. We were eighteen years old. We communicated telepathically, kept our legs intertwined, sinewy as the branches of a madrone.

Now I have to weigh everything: to call or not to call. To wait three days, five days, six. To ask everyone who might know him for information, to take this information and form a strategic plan. I shave my legs and my underarms, I make an appointment for a haircut, a manicure, all of which will make no difference if nothing is bound to happen. I don't know if anything will happen, but I plan for it anyway. I think about condoms, and blush, and wonder if he will buy any, wonder where they are in the store, how much they cost these days. I wonder about the weight of a man's hands on my shoulders, on my hair. Marilynne Robinson, in *Housekeeping*, writes that "need can blossom into all the compensations it requires.... To wish for a hand on one's hair is all but to feel it. So whatever we may lose, very craving gives it back to us again."

I want to believe her, so I crave the hand. I close my eyes and try to picture this man's wrists, to feel the soft underside of his wrist against my mouth. A man's wrists have always been the key to my lust; something rouses me in the power of a hand concentrated in that hinge. And yes, I feel it. Yes, my breath catches in my throat, as if he stroked his thumb against the edge of my jaw. My body's been so long without desire I've almost forgotten what it means to be a sexual being, to feel this quickening in my groin. And it's all I need for now: this moment of desire unencumbered by the complications of fulfillment. Because craving only gives rise to more craving; desire feeds on itself, and cannot be appeased. It is *my* desire after all, *my* longing, more delicious than realization, because over this longing I retain complete control.

I lied. I changed everything on my refrigerator, on my bulletin board, on my mantelpiece. I casually put up a picture, half-hidden, of myself on a good day, my tan legs long, my skin flawless as I pose in front of a blazing maple bush on Mill Creek. I try to suppress an unbidden fantasy: a photograph of me and this man and his two daughters filling in the empty place on my parents' wall. I know this is a dangerous and futile image, but it lodges anyway in my head.

I call my friend every half hour or so with updates on my frame of mind, asking for reassurance that I am not a terrible person. I ask questions as if she were a representative of the tourist board: "On what date does one start holding hands? Kissing? If I ask him out and he says yes, how do I know if he's just being polite?" If there were a phrasebook, I would buy it; a class, I would take it.

Yesterday I discussed this imminent dinner with my hairstylist, Tony, as he bobbed my hair. Tony has a new boyfriend, they're essentially married, but he's had his share of dating and he gives me both sides: "Well on the one hand, you've *got* to play the game," he says, waving the blow dryer away from my hair, "but on the other hand you need to show some honesty, some of the real you. You don't want to scare him off. This is a good lesson for you. Balance."

Tony is my guru. When I came to him the first time, a month after moving to Salt Lake City, I told him my hair was in a transition:

not long, not short, just annoying. "You can't think of it," said Tony, cupping my unwanted flip, "as a transition. This is what your hair wants to be right now. There are no transitions. This is *it*, right now."

Yesterday, he cupped my newly-coifed hair in his slender fingers, gazed at me somberly in the mirror. I smiled uncertainly, cocked my head. "Good?" he asked. "Good," I replied. He whisked bits of hair off my shoulders with a stiff brush. "Don't worry," he said. "Play it cool." I nodded, gazing at myself in the mirror which always makes my cheeks look a little too pudgy, my lips too pale. Whenever I look at myself too long, I become unrecognizable, my mouth slightly askew, a mouth I can't imagine kissing or being kissed. I paid Tony, then walked carefully out of the salon, my head level, a cold breeze against my bare neck. In the car, I did not resist the urge to pull down the rear-view mirror and look at myself again. I touched my new hair. I touched those lips, softly, with the very tips of my fingers.

A date. The word still brings up visions of Palm Springs, California and the date orchards on the outskirts of town, the sticky sweetness of the dark fruit. We drove through the orchards on car trips during the summers, my family hot and irritable in the blue station wagon. The stores had giant dates painted on their awnings, and when we stopped, our misery was forgotten. My mother doled the fruit out to us from the front seat, her eyes already half-closed in pleasure. The dates—heavy, cloying, dark as dried blood—always made the roof of my mouth itch, but I ate them anyway because they came in a white box like candy. I ate them because I was told they were precious, the food of the gods.

A man I like is coming to dinner. In two hours. The chicken is marinating, and the house is clean, and if I take a shower now and get dressed I'll have an hour and a half to sit fidgeting on my living room chair, talking to myself and to the fish, whose water, of course, I've changed. "Make a good impression," I plead with him. "Mellow out." He swims back and forth, avoiding my eyes, butting his pinhead against his bowl. I call my friend: Do I light candles? A fire in the fireplace? Do I use the cloth napkins? She says yes to the napkins, nix to everything else. I must walk the line between casual and serious, between cool and aflame. Perfume? Yes. Eyeliner? No. I remake the bed, only now realizing how misshapen my comforter is, all the feathers bunched into one end, so the coverlet lies forlornly against my pillows. It's yellowed at the edges, and my pillowcases are mismatched. Skirt or pants? I ask my friend. Wine or beer? My friend listens, a saint, then finally says: "Why are you asking me? I never get past the third date!" Suddenly I want to get off the phone as quickly as possible.

A man I like is coming to dinner. He's late. I sit on the edge of my bed, unwilling to stand near the front windows where he might see me waiting. My stomach hurts, and is not soothed by the smell of tandoori chicken overcooking in the oven. My hands, like a cliché, are sweating. I lie back on the bed, at this point not caring if I mess my hair, or wrinkle my green rayon dress, chosen for its apparent lack of effort. My name is painted in Japanese above my black bureau. Pieces of myself are scattered all around me: a blue kilim from Turkey, a seashell from Whidbey Island, a candlestick from Portugal. Pale light sifts through the venetian blinds at an angle just right for napping or making love. If I had to choose right now, I'd choose a nap, the kind that keeps me hovering on the edge of a consciousness so sweet it would seem foolish to ever resurface. My lavender eye pillow is within reach. My house is so small; how could it possibly accommodate a man, filling my kitchen chairs, peering at my refrigerator door?

On my bedside table is *The Pillow Book* of Sei Shonagan, a Japanese courtesan of the eleventh century, a woman whose career consisted in waiting. In this expectant state, she observed everything around her in great detail, found some of it to her liking and some not. I idly pick the book up and allow it to fall open. I read, "When a woman lives alone, her house should be extremely dilapidated, the mud wall should be falling to pieces, and if there is a pond, it should be overgrown with water plants. It is not essential that the garden be covered with sage-brush; but weeds should be growing through the sand in patches, for this gives the place a poignantly desolate look."

I close the book. I look around this apartment, this house where I live alone. My room feels clean, new, expectant. Now I want nothing more than to stay alone, to hold myself here in a state of controlled desire. But if this man doesn't show, I know my house will quickly settle into the dilapidation Shonagan saw fit for a single woman; the line between repose and chaos is thinner than I once thought. Despite all I've tried to learn in these years alone—about the worthiness of myself as an independent woman, about the intrinsic value of the present moment, about defining myself by my own terms, not by someone else's—despite all this, I know that my well-being this moment depends on a man's hand knocking on my door.

The doorbell rings, startling me into a sitting position. I clear my throat, which suddenly seems ready to close altogether, to keep me mute and safe. I briefly consider leaving the door unanswered; I imagine my date waiting, looking through the kitchen window, then backing away and into his car, shaking his head, wondering. Perhaps he would think me crazy, or dead. Perhaps he would call the police, tell them there's a woman he's worried about, a woman who lives alone. Or, more likely, he would drive to a bar, have a beer, forget about me. The thought of his absence momentarily pleases me, bathes me with relief. But of course I stand up and glance in the mirror, rake my hands through my hair to see it feather into place, and casually walk out to greet this man I like, this man who's coming to dinner.

Grape Hyacinths

HE TELLS ME HE USED TO DRINK THE DEW caught in the petals of grape hyacinths lining the road to his grade school in Montana. I say: *that must be why you're a poet,* and he smiles up at me from the grass, strokes his hand against the hyacinths spilling against my porch. He leans down and puts his lips against the buds, mimes for me the sip, his eyes closing as he drinks.

There are many words we've yet to say to one another, this man and I, words unfamiliar and awkward in our mouths. As I watch him, I feel these words rise in my throat and beat there, a faint pulse. *Come here,* he says, *you have to put your nose right in them,* and so I kneel with him on the lawn, bending to these untamed weeds. The buds at the tip are tight and round, like small fruits of the currant bush, a grape that grows in the rising light of Corinth. Down the stalk, the inflorescence fans open into lace-edged bells. I press my cheek against their flesh, inhale the scent of distant vineyards, the evaporated dew. I smell *Muscari*, the family of musk from which these buds descend. They yield against my lips like a kiss.

It's spring in Salt Lake City, and I can't seem to budge more than a few feet from my porch; I want to be here when the Japanese cherry peaks; I want to keep smelling the violets, the incipient iris. Behind me, in a circle dug into the lawn, blue tulips stand like chalices of lavender glass. They seduce me into staying put, their tongues fluent in the endless dusk. When I touch them, their pollen simmers on my fingers. I remember planting them last fall, burying the bulbs beneath the pansies, surprised I would perform an act committing me to one place. *Blue tulips*, I said to myself then, and wondered if they would really arrive, if they would be blue, if they would last more than a day. It's been a week now and they keep speaking, telling me to stay, to stay, to stay. Landscaping trucks appear, white and flecked with gold; like strange migratory birds, they circle the neighborhood.

We're drinking sake, the poet and I. We're watching the last of the day flood across my lawn. I don't know if I'll stay forever, but we're on our knees in the grape hyacinths, drinking wine made from grains of rice, and this seems like enough for now. I'd like to imagine us in Japan, in the spring, saluting the cherry blossoms with small, ceramic cups. I imagine us in cotton kimonos, after the bath, sipping the dew from each other's skin, articulate with words no longer foreign to our tongues.

Time With Children

3:14 A.M. I SIT IN THE KITCHEN and listen to the rest of the house asleep. Eight-year-old Hannah sprawls on the living-room carpet with no pillow, no blanket—she seems all limbs, sleek and toned as an expensive colt. I've covered her with a quilt, which somehow makes her position more acceptable, more like sleep. Sarah, four, snores like a small, wild animal: her mouth open, her body skewed in its Pocahontas pajamas. In this apartment the girls have no bedroom of their own; they make do with the convertible sofa in the front room. They love the transformation of sofa into bed and often fight with each other over who will be responsible for this most mundane of acts. Their father, in his bedroom, in the bed I've just left, snores in harmony with Sarah; they echo each other, his drone transforming hers into something more sonorous, more adult. His alarm is set for 5:17, and I know when it goes off Joel will hit the snooze button twice before rising.

And so this family sleeps all around me, each person joined to the other inside the muted phases of the night. I know Joel recreates his daughters even in his sleep, that language makes them new to him; again and again the girls arrive in his poems: lovely bodies, fresh, always transcendent. I know Sarah and Hannah sometimes sleep-walk into their father's room at night, bumping their way back to his body through instinct. But I don't know where I fit in this con-stellation, how to define myself even as I sit in this kitchen chair, in the heart of the house. These girls are not my daughters, not my step-daughters; I have no word for them, no name to adequately describe our relationship. "My boyfriend's girls," I sometimes say, which fails to satisfy me because it puts the "boyfriend" first, solidifies his role as intermediary. Or my "little friends," but this phrase trivializes them, fails to describe how fully alive I feel in their presence and yet how dull, how lugubrious, watching as they lurch their way in the world. Here I am, a nameless sentinel in the private hours, prowling among their vulnerable bodies in the dark.

Sarah expects the world to love her and it does. Hannah is wise already, knows love's part of a greater exchange, sets her mouth and watches first. Now, in their sleep, their bodies have abandoned all pretense, all the fight of getting what they need and want. In a few hours I'll wake these girls and begin getting them ready for school. I'll fix them Lucky Charms and hot chocolate, pack their lunches with thin bologna sandwiches and cups of sweetened yogurt. I'll get them dressed, try to brush their hair, get them in the car, drive them to two different schools. Sarah might forget her blanket and she'll cry when we get to Montessori, twist away from me in the backseat and scream until I have to forcibly drag her from the car. A mother will pass me in the parking lot, murmur "a rough start?" and I'll nod knowingly, as if I'm an expert in such things, an old hand.

But I'm no such thing. I'm a novice, an impostor. These girls usually live with their mother during the school year; I'm filling in for a crisis. Their mother now goes to the "House of Hope" twelve hours a day, a place of recovery for alcoholics and drug addicts. Joel has told me stories about their marriage, about the vodka bottles found stashed in the shoe bin, the mornings he couldn't wake her, the screaming fights in the house near the cemetery. She's a pretty woman, with a beautiful voice; I once saw her on stage at the Opera House, singing Beethoven's "Ode to Joy" with the Salt Lake City Chorus. Through my binoculars I watched her throat open wide for the exultant notes, her eyes bright with concentration as they focused on the conductor. But just last week, when we stopped by her apartment early to pick up Hannah's violin, her voice wavered and broke as she thanked me for taking care of her children. Her eyes were red, stretched thin around the edges. I averted my gaze, mumbled something about how it was my pleasure, no problem, don't worry about it.

The first day Sarah rolled under the bed and refused to come out. I knelt on the rug and twisted my head to find her flattened beneath the cushions. "I can't do this, Sarah," I said, emphasizing each word, trying to put some authority in my voice, and Hannah, laughing beside me on the floor, said, "That's because you're not a mom."

I'll drive back across town thirty minutes in rush hour traffic to retrieve Sarah's blanket, and still I won't be a Mom; I'll fetch it back to her classroom where she'll be sitting at a small table by herself, eating Trix out of a baggie. She will take the blanket from me with no surprise or gratitude, settle herself into her customary position, with the corner of the blanket wedged firmly between her front teeth. She'll flash me a smile, currency she knows stretches far. I'll feel a swell of righteous anger, then let it go. By now I've realized what most parents have known all along: the value of surrender, the necessity of such concession when spending time with children.

By the end of it I'm exhausted, but oddly grounded and calm, in a way that fifteen years of meditation practice has never taught me. I've spent days, weeks, months sitting on meditation cushions and watching my breath. I've created perfectly quiet environments, with incense and bells, in which to contemplate the impermanence of all existence. I've walked silently around the perimeter of meditation retreats, my hands neatly clasped beneath my heart. But nothing has forced me into the present moment as much as these mornings with two young girls.

Now, in these weeks when I'm a pseudo-mom, I come home to my empty house and it no longer feels empty, just mine, and quiet. I feel no twinge of panic, no lingering questions as to my purpose, my validity. I just make coffee, go out on my front porch, feel the air turning toward autumn, and think about Hannah in her new blue dress saying good-bye to Sarah as if she would never see her again. I'll worry about her, and this worry will make me feel necessary. I'll begin forgetting the overturned chocolate milk, the tangled hair, the messy house and remember only child bodies brushing against me, trusting without calculation.

3:49 A.M. I know I'll stay awake now till dawn. There's a keening beneath my skin out of synch with the crickets, with the breath-sleep of those around me. The room smells vaguely of last night's dinner—Sloppy Joes on sesame buns—food I never would have considered before spending time with children, but last night I loved it: the sweet-salty tang of the meat, the sponginess of the bread. The refrigerator rattles to a halt, and silence pulses through the house.

The windows still frame only the night, and I know at some point all things will take on their proper outlines: the swing in the cherry tree, the railing on the deck, the chain link of the tennis court next door. I want to stay awake and catch the moment when the world becomes unambiguous and clear, but I know it will elude me again: I'll blink at the wrong time, or be preoccupied with other things.

On the kitchen table there's an anthology of poetry edited by Czeslaw Milosz: *A Book of Luminous Things*. I pick it up and there, between the pages, I find a white sheet of paper, instructions from the Mormon Handicrafts Guild on how to knit bandages for Leper/ Tropical Sores. It tells me I must "use the knit stitch all around for the proper give." It states that "white or muslin are the proper colors, but flesh color can also be used." This list of instructions startles me, and I picture children with open sores, holding their arms out to be bandaged; I picture myself wrapping hand-knit bandages around the stumps of an infant's legs. The instructions, forgotten by an anonymous Mormon woman who most likely had many children vying for her attention, are folded between the leaves of two poems in the book. In one of these, a young woman "...finds herself before/a mirror with worm eaten frame/she contemplates in it her virgin torso...." In the other, "when he pressed his lips to my mouth/the knot fell open of itself...."

The body and its extremes. Bodies transparent with longing and desire. Bodies scoured with disease, bandaged by religious hands. The conjunction of the two is what makes for luminosity—desire on the edge of decay. The children walk this rim all the time: their bodies making and unmaking themselves moment to moment. It seems fitting to me that a woman who knits bandages for people deemed "untouchable" would, in a free moment, pick up this book of poems, read the verses, hold both extremes of the body simultaneously in her competent hands.

4:22 A.M. My skin, in the light from the thrift-store lamp, looks pale, loose along the ankles, and I can see my mother's veins spidering up my calf. I'm turning into an old woman, here in this night without sleep; I'm losing the chance to remake myself, as the children do each night.

After I take the girls to school this morning, I'll go to Emma's house. Emma is six months old, and I think she loves me. I'm her nanny, but what is she to me, what shall I call her? Again, as with Hannah and Sarah, I have no name for her, no label to validate our relationship, no way to clearly situate myself in a world that still expects a woman to marry, to have her own children clinging to her side.

When I arrive at Emma's house, it will be almost time for her afternoon nap. She'll be happy to see me; she'll give me her tooth-less smile, her new sounds. Always, when I stare at her, I can't help but repeat her name. I stamp *Emma* on her with my lips; I say *Emma* to the bottoms of her feet, to the curlicue of her ear, to the belly button still ripe with the cord. She, in turn, clutches my hair, maneuvers my head back so she can read my lips, know her name, and through this name remember whole-body love, this love that knows no bounds, not yet.

At home, I have a photograph by Julia Margaret Cameron: *The Kiss of Peace*. A young woman, her eyes lidded with sorrow, brushes a kiss onto a child's forehead. They are both shrouded in muslin, their hair long and disheveled, their faces muddied as if they've just come in from a storm. The woman's lips barely touch the child's skin; it is an absent gesture, one made in weariness and habit. It could be any kiss, on any day, barely noticed. My eyes are drawn again and again to the place where the woman's lips brush the child's forehead, to the point of contact that could so easily be missed.

We go through our days like this, absently touching each other, especially the children. And perhaps that's the point of this photograph, taken by a woman who raised ten children, who wrote 300 letters a month, who ran her husband's household in India and took up photography as a hobby: that any moment of contact, however brief, is equivalent to a kiss of peace, a gesture whose design is holy.

5:15 A.M. I am awake in the most unexpected hour, when sprinklers come on automatically, and children sigh, and Joel hits the snooze button on the clock radio, the numbers luminous in the dark room, the only light coming from the clicking of time, the changing over. To myself, I count the children I will care for today, as if they were eggs I collect in the morning. Emma, Sarah, and Hannah—the three of them like gradated illustrations of childhood. I feel like an adult finally, installed unequivocally in the adult world. Because of this, I think about all the things that could go wrong: falls from the crib, errant cars at intersections, illness. And then I let them go, staying in my Zen parent mode, at peace with the fact that I have no idea what the next moment will bring.

But I know, if I were a *real* parent, this attitude could never last; serenity can take you only so far. I remember the framed poster my mother kept on her kitchen counter: "Worry is the advance interest we pay on troubles that seldom come." Even now, I see her meditating on this phrase, trying to smooth the permanent anxiety etched into her forehead. If I were a real parent, if there were no finite end to this responsibility, no cease to the extravagant claims these children make on me, I know my calm would gradually erode. I don't think I could do it: be a mom, situated forever on the brink of unspeakable despair.

I remember, years ago, when I first heard about the bombing of the Federal Building in Oklahoma City. I was staying by myself at Rhea's house in the Mendocino hills, and I switched on NPR as an antidote to all that quiet. I heard something about a bombing, something about many of the dead being small children. I looked out at my friend's forsythia bush swaying in the wind. I refocused my gaze on the flat leaves of the bay tree tapping against the glass. I heard about the bodies they were just then finding in the rubble, the firemen carrying out charred infants and toddlers.

I sat there listening for I don't know how long, my hand pressed tightly to my mouth. Finally I went out on the porch to sit with the dog. I sat with one hand on his neck, petting and petting, while rain blew into my face and my hair; rain bent the rosebushes and the delphinium. Through the closed door I could still hear the voices on the radio, the murmur of a community repairing itself through bits of information. And I couldn't help it: I imagined myself as one of the mothers, arriving at the building, searching for my child. The sense of it was so strong, I felt myself flush with panic. I saw the children laid out on the ground, felt myself stumbling toward them.

And then I came back to myself, back to California and the rain that trickled steadily into the apple trees, the Asian pear, the peaches. And I felt, I admit, a flood of guilty relief that I was not a parent, that I would never have to look for my own dead child among the debris of a disaster.

At the same time, I knew I was implicated. The children in Oklahoma City *were* my children, as they would become everybody's children in the days to come. The pictures would arrive with astonishing swiftness. We would open the papers, see the photographs, read the names. We would cry in our cars, listening to the radio. We would look over at a stoplight and see others crying in their cars as well, their hands still clutching the steering wheel, but this anonymous camaraderie in the face of tragedy will not be enough to redeem it.

I got up from the bench; the dog shook himself and ran off into the rain. I went back inside. The house was sheltered by hundreds of trees, all of them green and vivid with leaves. I could turn to them now for solace if I chose, see their reverberant life as some bitter compensation for loss. But I saw the trees as only themselves, seeding and spawning because that's what trees do. I turned off the radio and listened to the silence settle on me, a blanket of fine dust, the cloth of all my days come to claim me.

5:28 A.M. and the world rises to meet me, to coincide; I hear a slither of bedclothes, a chorus of sighs. I wait for them all to wake, to find me already here in the morning without them. I wait for their startled faces, their surprise at my presence.

When we first meet children, we often ask two questions: "What is your name?" and "How old are you?" The more difficult questions come later; for now these two suffice as an overture for communication. The children often do not speak but hold up their hands, signing to us with their fingers: two, four, or six. When I first met Sarah she was learning sign language in preschool; she signed to me her name, her hands clenching and unclenching, her face furrowed in concentration. Weeks later she came to me and her hands twisted at her heart, traversed the space between us to turn at my own. *I love you. You love me.* At times her whole body is the sign for love, and I nod my head *Yes, oh yes.*

Sunlight glides across the back lawn. In a few hours I'll drive the girls to school, and this same sun will glare in my eyes, dangerous, and I won't be able to see the oncoming cars; I'll be blind, working off intuition alone. I'll make sure everyone is buckled up, and even as I do so I'll feel an unreasonable pride at the small bodies in my car, the way their heads in the windows give my vehicle importance, weight, destination. I'll inch my way into the intersection, and pray.

A Field Guide
to the Desert

I. Grand Wash

A wash, in the desert, is a dry place defined by water. Not water flowing, but the memory of water's flow. In the car, with the children, you point out the window and name rock formations as they slither by: *Chimney Rock, The Castle, Fiery Furnace.* The girls sit up straight but keep eating their Doritos, quickly moving hand to mouth, as if there won't be enough. Their mother, you know, hardly eats anymore; she sits at the kitchen table and perhaps drinks vodka from water glasses, her throat so dry nothing will quench her thirst. She's become brittle and a little blurred around the edges. She no longer attends the "House of Hope"; perhaps hope, for her, no longer has a dwelling place, a doorway to enter. Soon she will lose custody of the girls; you all know this, but have not yet said the words or drawn up the complicated papers. She's too tired to help the girls pack, so their suitcases reveal an odd assortment of winter clothes and bathing suits, tartan sweaters, and sundresses made of rayon.

Their father rarely looks at you as he drives. He keeps the music turned up a tad too loud, and bends his ear toward you when you speak. You and he haven't touched now in a long time, but you remember how, when you first made love, you felt your body grow dark and light at the same time, a shadowed canyon livid with secrets. You remember the tip of his tongue on your tongue, the apex of his hip against yours, a circle of flesh and bone. You remember the girls asleep in the room next to yours, how this made you furtive, discreet. You extinguished all the lights, so that you knew each other only through touch. You memorized each other this way, your hands passing over flesh and bone in the dark.

The children ask a lot of questions that begin with "why." You think how improbable they are, these girls—drops of flesh drawn by a strange gravity to take hold in this world. Tell them: you can't understand the desert from afar. You have to get inside and touch your face to the rock.

When you dare to hike up the canyon with no name, even the children grow quiet. They dig their hands beneath the sand until they're trapped like animals and struggle to move, laughing silently, their eyes wide on yours. You think about the bodies they've come from—their mother, her body so damaged it seems no more than carapace. You think about their father and his body you once stroked so reverently, thinking *this* is what marriage means: guarding the bodies that muster children within them.

Sarah looks up at you with her mother's face, grinning. Hannah climbs the wall, waves down at you, her arms long, slender and brown—arms that bear no precedent. You no longer have peripheral vision but circular vision, seeing what's beside you, behind you, in front. You're caught by the smallest red leaf crenellated on the silver-twigged sage, and then next to it the crimson start of Indian paintbrush, and the sand next to your knee: see how it's made of sixteen different rocks, the facets of them now so small, so even, they please you in a way no human hand ever will again.

When you finally walk away, the canyon tugging at your back like a fretful mother, you'll see the girls' father from a distance, see his eyes on you and his daughters, countering the undertow of the canyon, pulling the three of you toward him with his gaze. Your eyesight will be so clear, so sharp, you can see flecks of gold, like mica, in his iris. That night, you know, you'll want to touch him again, feel his body yield under your hand, caving in.

It's snowing in the desert. This weather seems impossible, but the snowflakes don't think so. They light on the girls' hair, on their shoulders, as you meander out the canyon, your bodies scrubbed clean by sand. The snow makes a beaded curtain that seals up the canyon behind you, holding you inside it, already translucent, like a memory.

II. Cassidy Arch

You'll sit with the children on the slickrock above an arch that seems not so much arch but bridge, and not bridge but DANGER, DANGER. You'll sit out of the wind, eating peanut butter and honey sandwiches, and though you won't touch the girls, every fiber of your body leans toward them—to keep them here, away from the edge, your arm ready to swing out and pin them against the rock. Keep your gaze focused on the small things right in front of you: Sarah's boot, one lace dangling and damp; Hannah's lips working around her sandwich; the dirty knife askew on a ledge so smooth it could be glass. The three of you wait for the father, who is lost, to find you. At some point you'll allow the children to stand up and peer over the edge while you hold on to their coats.

You huddle again in the arms of the rock. You look back on the slickrock trail, that is not a trail but a route, marked with cairns that merge now into an expanse of high desert. There is no way home. You'll become hungry when the food runs out; you'll eat juniper berries and prickly pear, working your lips around the thorns like a small, starving marmot.

Sarah climbs on your lap and holds her face so close to yours it becomes the entire world, and the world smells of peanut butter and girl and the coming snow. Hannah spots the witch's nipple, the peak by which you navigated on the way up. *So we're not lost,* she says. *We're here.* In the distance you see the blue shimmer of their father's parka. He's found you. You're not an animal after all.

III. Sulfur Creek

It's not exactly walking *on* water you want, but it could be. Anyone looking from afar would see it as so, your feet below the water, your bodies upright, infused with a light that could be godly. In the Sea of Galilee, they're building a transparent bridge two inches beneath the surface, so the tourists can walk there and be Jesus a while. As if the posture is all it takes to be transformed.

It's not a trail, but a route, the ranger warned you, but there's no way to get lost. The creek provides. You must cross and recross, your shoes no longer shoes but sponges, and the children are hungry for more of it; they refuse, now, to walk anywhere dry. When you get to the waterfall, the children scramble up the rock, arms and legs akimbo, and look down at you, laughing. You jump and fall, the stone set against you, but finally you make it in your bare feet, your toes painted an opalescent pink that looks both strange and lovely against the desert. The current runs faster now, goaded by the narrow canyon.

The sky is clear and hot. Snow is no longer a thought. Water babbles underneath the blooming tamarisks, the trees Willa Cather loved. "They looked, indeed, like very old posts," she wrote, "well seasoned and polished by time, miraculously endowed with the power to burst into delicate foliage and flowers, to cover themselves with long brooms of lavender-pink blossom...." One tamarisk stretches up the red wall of the canyon, casual in its blossom, waving in every direction at once.

You walk upriver until there's a cave, an overhang of rock. Part of you wants to dry in the sun, while part of you wants to sleep in the shade. You do both, while the children wander too near the river and back. Their father will hold their hands, or wrap his thumb and forefinger around their wrists. The voices come closer and recede. There's no need to say it: danger shimmers beneath the surface of all lovely things.

IV. Goblin Valley

The children want to become rock. They scatter among the goblins, find the deepest holes, the smallest cracks in which to disappear. You scramble up to a cave and sit there like small animals waiting out the heat of the day. Kneeling on bare rock, they call you to look at the "tiny handprints!" they've found. You imagine red Anasazi handprints on varnished walls, the fingerprints of an infant as ancient birth record on the rock. But you see, in the sand, the tiny footprints of an animal—a chipmunk perhaps? a prairie dog?— and you imagine his dark eyes on you, his whiskers twitching, as he waits for the danger to pass.

You see a couple hiking barefoot on the gray rock. There's nothing here to harm them. They hold hands, laughing, and run up the canyon as if advertising soft drinks. You ask the children if they want to take off their shoes, but they blush as if you've asked them to strip naked and dance. They keep walking, their shoes on, their canteens swinging and dripping against their thighs.

You want them to drink water, more than they're willing, to keep their bodies liquid, not rock. You want them, when they go home, to find their mother alive and well, her body restored, the vodka bottles discarded in favor of bread, whole chickens, soup. You want their father to love you, to give you a reason to stay. You want to be animal tracks on their skin, so light they won't notice when you're gone.

V. Salt Lake City

When you get back to Salt Lake City, the girls' mother is not well. You see her out the corner of your eye as you unload the car, and to you it's like watching a face dissolve, a horse in terror, the skin around her eyes pulled back and white. She passes you on the stairs, crying, her arms angular as twigs. Sarah looks at you, says, "See you next week?" and you say, "Yes, sweetheart, see you." She turns, and you watch her climb the steps, carrying her canteen and hiking boots in her arms. Hannah leaves the car in silence. Her body looks too tired, suddenly, for a child, too small to carry the weight of her head.

You watch them go, and you do not cry out to stop them, you do not fling your arm across their bodies, though the danger is clear, clearer than on the precipice of Cassidy Arch. You say not a word. You make only a little scrabbling noise in your throat, like a small animal scratching its way toward water, toward food.

Gourd

THE GOURD SPEAKS TO ME OF SEED, of what remains when flesh no longer fits to the bone. When I take it in my hand I expect the gourd to speak of the summer, of what transpired underground before it began to climb. Who knows? These gardens are well-tended in the desert, the gardeners so considerate of the gourds. They irrigate them with hoses thin as veins. They build trellises so the gourds, when they fruit, sway high off the ground, like the biblical gourd of Jonah that rose in the night and shaded the man as he learned about forgiveness.

The gardeners build huts, dark and cool, for the gourds to rest in when they're done. They stroke their gourds and speak to each other of seed for the seasons to come. They argue over methods: whether to scrape the skin while green, or wait until the fruit is dry, mottled, and aching to be peeled. They prop the most voluptuous gourds in their windows—some with necks haughty as swans, some of them the yellow of butter, others pale as milk. The gourds lean toward one another, as if whispering of the old days.

My gourd tilts against the window next to my bed, cocking its long neck, eyeing me like a question mark. It smells, vaguely, of cocoa, as if the ground it grew in were fertilized with chocolate. I expect it be warm, but when I lift it to my cheek, the skin is cool and smooth as what I imagine my heart to be, these mornings before I leave for good. I expect, when I'm gone, I'll remember these mornings as free of desire, my body full of bones still dense, resting comfortably in their sockets. When I'm far from the desert, in a place where water is not a question, I know I'll want heat and bare rock and fruit that grows hollow and light. I'll hold the gourd in my lap and watch rain fall outside my window, beating the sky into a rumpled sheet. I know I'll want the glassy face of the desert looking back at me. I'll want the side canyon whose questions are clear and come with answers that take only time, and more time, to answer.

The gardeners tell me I can make of my gourd an instrument. I can drill a small hole and fill it with seed. I can balance it on my palms and tilt it one way, then the other, so it makes a babble like rain. I can listen and listen, until it sounds to me like rock making its way back to sand.

Kimono

CERTAIN SUMMER MORNINGS, LIKE THIS ONE, I like to put on a kimono that came from Japan. It's cut from a sturdy white cotton, with red vines trailing across the folds. I like the triangular sleeves that suspend in points from the elbow; they lend to each gesture of my arms an elegance missing from the rest of my dutiful wardrobe. The narrow belt has no loops to anchor it, so I overlap the panels in front and tie them firmly against me with a flat knot.

I wear this robe only when I'm alone, on mornings when I have time to gaze out into the distance and settle into a good bout of melancholy. I hold my coffee cup to my lips with both hands, and assume a Matisse-like pose, all line and gesture, a sketch titled: "Woman, Solo Again." The belt nestles into my hipbones, and I feel held, swaddled, contained.

I know this type of robe may not properly be called a kimono in Japan; I know that word might be reserved for the silky dress of the geisha, not a word to be thrown around with careless abandon. I'm sure my boyfriend of many years ago, Keith, taught me the correct name for this garment; he was a man who liked precision in language and would frown now if he could hear me; he would shake his head quickly, already rising from his seat, his lips slightly parted to correct me. I don't mean to portray him as mean-spirited; he was a man generous with knowledge, and often with love. He had brought this robe back with him from Japan, as a present for his father's mother, a woman we called "Gram."

He gave the kimono to me on the day of his grandmother's funeral. The rest of the family stayed in the front room of her house, while Keith and I slipped into her bedroom together. The autumn light had gone silver through the windowpane, and all her things lay still as she left them: the bureau with the family photographs in pewter frames, the book on the night stand, the quilt smooth on the bed. We stepped inside, opened her closet door, and I recalled the first time I'd seen Gram wearing the kimono. She had taken the robe from a hanger and slipped her arms through those voluminous sleeves. Gram always reminded me of a sandpiper: those same spindly limbs, but with a compact energy that shimmered all along her body. Her head came up only to my breastbone; she always seemed to tilt forward, eager to go somewhere, anywhere, as long as it was with you. As she wrapped the kimono around her waist, the folds of it fell in graceful pleats down to the wood floor. She tied the belt in a neat square knot, held out her arms to the side and smiled. The bright red vines brought out the color in her powdery cheeks; her small feet pointed outward with a ballerina's poise. She stood there, her arms flaring from her sides like wings, awaiting our response.

A robe is such an intimate gift to give a woman. One can't help but imagine the fabric bending to the woman's body, covering her nakedness after the bath. It is a gesture both innocent and touching—

this desire to cover and protect and make warm. I looked at Gram standing there, wrapped in a robe from a country she would never dream of seeing, and I think I understood, fleetingly, the quality of love that can transpire between grandmothers and grandchildren, the kind of love that families, no matter how complex, are designed to sanctify.

"Beautiful!" I cried, and Keith clapped his hands, and Gram nodded shyly, and began unwinding the kimono from around her waist. She turned spindly again as she emerged from this wrapper. She hung the robe back up very carefully and put it away; I doubt she ever wore it again. Perhaps she felt it was too "good" for everyday wear; it was more of a sacrament, a token of her grandson's devotion. One doesn't wear such love everyday; one must keep it whole, untarnished, under wraps.

Years ago, Keith and I lived in a tiny attic apartment off First Street in Missoula, Montana. Actually Keith lived there; I was merely a frequent visitor to those rooms with their buttery wood paneling, the ceilings that sloped down sharply to the eaves. It could have been claustrophobic but really it was a chamber out of a fairy tale, with a double bed tucked into one dormer, a breakfast nook in the other, the couch and coffee table dead center against the front wall. Everything had its place and fit there with remarkable charm. I remember cooking tandoori chicken in the tiny kitchen, or fish curries, or big bowls of potato salad to go with the elk sausage our landlord sometimes dropped at our door. It grew outrageously hot in that apartment, so in the summer we often ate outside on the deck and watched bicyclists make their way down to the Clark Fork River.

When we talked about moving to Vermont to live with Gram, it was with the wistful countenance of children planning an afternoon excursion. Gram needed companionship; her small town was quiet and promised endless hours of solitude and writing time. We wouldn't need much money. We would eat lots of maple syrup and homemade jams. We could get Ben & Jerry's ice cream whenever we wanted. There was at least one good restaurant in the town—it served a succulent and meaty pot roast—and one health food store. It might be good for us, we thought, a change of pace from Western life, where people strung up antelopes in the garage during hunting season.

Gram had asked us to come to Vermont because she hated to be alone. It's true she had a housemate, Geraldine, who lived on the main floor of the house; her rooms seemed much more spacious than Gram's, full as they were with antiques and cupboards of crystal and photo albums with embroidered sleeves. Geraldine and Gram had settled into a cozy familiarity in the twenty years they had lived together, but they seemed to have little intimacy beyond the arguments over grocery bills and postage stamps.

Gram, who had only one son and a husband long dead, hungered for family. Family was the only thing that seemed to give her sustenance. She always mourned the passing of summer; on the Fourth of July she'd sigh and say, "Summer's almost over," already missing the visits with her son and grandchildren, the warm nights that allowed her to breathe easily in her sleep.

So that summer we took a reconnaissance visit to her town, ate the pot roast in that diner, scoped out the quaint, rundown buildings on Main Street. The second morning, early, I woke in the dark to Gram faintly calling out Keith's name, in a voice strangled with panic. I heard her wheezing chest, the terrible catch in her throat. Keith still slept, and I nudged him. *"Go,"* I whispered. He rose from our bed and, still half asleep, carried her downstairs. I stumbled behind, carrying clothing and coats.

We rushed her to the E.R. and waited many hours (could it have been an entire day? It seems now that it was almost dark again when we took her out the exit doors). Keith and I watched a John Wayne western in its entirety on the small, ceiling-mounted television in the waiting room. We sat slumped in the orange plastic chairs, our backs and heads aching, grumpily holding Styrofoam cups of coffee. We barely spoke at all; perhaps I rubbed his shoulders, perhaps not. Yet, still, when Gram appeared, holding gingerly to the elbow of a nurse, we stood up and greeted her with wide smiles and open arms, as if we'd just spend the most pleasant day of a renewing vacation.

"You two are getting *pot roast* tonight!" she said, with such emphasis there was no arguing with her, and we went to the diner and ate their pot roast again, though this time, the meat and potatoes seemed not quite as succulent, and I could see that this dish might prove poor fare if eaten too often. They called it Yankee Pot Roast, I think now, because one ate it in the presence of all those stalwart Yankees, Northerners to the bone. They wore flannel shirts and twill pants that gave off an odor of maple sugar and hay; their hair was cut neatly around the ears. Gram hardly ate any pot roast herself, but she watched our faces, hoping the food would be enough to keep us in Vermont, to keep us with her.

In the end, Keith and I decided against Vermont—too cold in the winter, too isolated—and it turned out not to matter because in early November Gram died of emphysema. The call came from his father, early in the morning, and we let the machine pick up. We had been to a Halloween party the night before, a loud and liquid affair, where all the women, including me, wore red lipstick bright as blood. Keith had drunk too much, and I had watched him weave between the men and women, his eyes too bright, the hair at the nape of his neck damp. We'd come home grumpy and gone to bed without saying a word. On the machine we heard his father's voice. "Gram passed on late last night. Call me." We heard this voice as we lay in that bed by the window, and Keith moaned, rolled over to face the wall.

I called his father back. I said the initial words of sympathy and consolation *("I'm so sorry; she was such a wonderful woman...")*. As I think of it now, I remember him telling me he stayed with Gram in the end, that he watched her worn-out chest rise and fall. I saw him as a child: an adult child, but performing a child's most hallowed task. Even now I can imagine the gray room, lit faintly by the street lamp outside, the high bed covered with a light-blue quilt. Gram's body makes hardly a ripple in those covers, so slight she's become, so faint. I see the low chair in which Terry keeps watch. I see neither of their faces, only the silhouettes of their bodies, their heads. What's more clear is the connection that binds them together, now in this room, at the moment of departure. A son. A mother. Familial love like oxygen in the room; time measured out breath by shuddering breath. I wonder if his own breath caught in his throat, if he rose a little out of his chair to catch sight of that last inhalation.

But surely this memory of mine, this dramatic scene, cannot be correct. Terry, a reticent man, would not have confided such things in me, even if they were true. We must have spoken only as much as necessary to make the arrangements, while Keith directed me from the bed, his voice garbled, his hands covering his eyes. I made chicken soup and called the airlines, pretending to be married in order for both of us to get the bereavement fares, which were still too high, over $800 for each of us. I talked to his father again, who said he would pay for both of us to come.

He wanted me to be there, he said. He said I was part of the family.

We left for Vermont early the next day, flying in a prop plane out of Missoula. Keith brought his laptop computer on the plane and began to compose Gram's eulogy, squinting at the screen in the low, flickering light. I could already imagine how he would structure it: Keith was a fiction writer, a good one, and I knew he would begin the eulogy by describing the circumstances of Gram's birth, then go on to describe how that inauspicious beginning marked the kind of person she eventually became.

He would tell how Gram was born in a rural farmhouse in the dead of winter during a flu epidemic. Her father died the day after she was born; her mother died a few days later. Keith would evoke the flickering darkness of that house, the twin odors of birth and death, the faceless siblings milling about the infant born practically an orphan. There were too many children in that house already, all of them now motherless, so her older sister wrapped the baby in a multitude of shawls and brought her in a horse-drawn buggy, in a blizzard, over the Vermont hills to live with relatives. Gram, herself, had often related the next part of the story to me, her voice lowered as if telling of forbidden things: they stop by the side of the road for some reason (to rest the horses? to check a map?), and the sister peeks at the newborn in her swaddling clothes. And she's not breathing. Not a sound, not a peep, no movement at all in the chest or the mouth.

As the sister watches, horrified, poking the baby in the chest, the child takes one long shuddering in-breath and decides to remain in the world. But in that world she feels always an outsider, living with an aunt and uncle, running up to the windows of the village church but never going inside: this is the picture I know Keith will make of

Gram in his eulogy. A woman who never felt fully at home, who knew she was here by the faintest providence. A woman who always had trouble catching her breath, never trusting fully that the next breath would come.

Terry had found us rooms at a motel near the funeral home; when we walked in I saw our room had mirrors all along the wall, creating a montage of reflections. As soon as his father left, Keith brushed the hair away from my neck and kissed my shoulder, in the exact spot that made me weak in the knees. He reached around and undid one button of my shirt, then another. I watched this in the mirror, then took his hands and lifted them away from me. "No, we're here for a funeral," I said, in the prim voice I'd come to use more and more frequently with him, a voice full of peevishness and thwarted expectations. It was the voice of a woman near the end of a relationship, traveling as a fake wife in a falsified marriage. But it would still be years before either of us could understand such things, so we merely turned away from our full-length reflections to unpack our bags, both of us silently seething.

This was the first funeral I'd ever attended. My grandfather had died when I was twelve, but none of us were asked to accompany my mother to the funeral; my father stayed home and cared for me and my brothers while my mother went to sit *shiva* with her mother, covering the mirrors in black cloth. She told me this when she called home, her voice distant and sticky with grief. An adult cousin of mine had died under mysterious circumstances (suicide?) when I was seven or eight, but we weren't allowed to the funeral, only to the house afterward for the food and commiseration. One friend of mine had died in college, jumping off the roof of his dormitory at UCLA while tripping for the first time on LSD, but for some reason none of us were invited to that funeral, or else we felt so guilty for allowing him up on that roof in the first place that we shied away from facing his family.

So I had never actually seen a coffin, or mourners, or bodies dressed for burial. That night, along with Keith's sister, Amy, we went to the mortuary for the viewing. Perhaps I expected to sit and look at a varnished coffin, the corpse decently stowed away, out of sight. But when we walked into the parlor, there was Gram, propped up in her casket, wearing the only good dress she owned: a cornflower-blue silk sprinkled with roses and peonies. This dress had shown up in every family portrait for years. It had a tiny white bow tied neatly at the apex of her collarbone. Her glasses sat on the bridge of her nose, a little too tightly, as if they would leave two red marks when she took them off to sleep.

I think it startled all of us: the son, the grandchildren, as we filed into the room. I could feel all of us balk for just a half-stride before continuing our baleful procession. I had never seen a body so still, her frame now mere mannequin for the dress in which she'd taken such pride. I wasn't sure what to do so I watched Amy kneel by the coffin and hold a rose quartz heart between her palms for a moment, in a gesture of prayer. She then placed it solemnly on her grandmother's breast, and leaned in to kiss Gram lightly on the forehead. Amy is an actress, and I could see her calculating each of these moves before she made them, but the kiss took me by surprise, seemed to surprise Amy herself who hurriedly stood up and twirled away from the coffin and back to the foyer. Terry stood grimly in a black suit and then backed off from the coffin to speak with the mortician.

I wish I could remember exactly Keith's gestures as he stood next to his grandmother. I think he wept as he covered her hand with his, but I can't say for sure. I do know he looked handsome in his dark suit (he always did; suits emphasized his square shoulders and the lifeguard "V" he spent hours at the gym sculpting), and I felt repentant for my earlier rebuff. I stood a little to the side as he bent stiffly over the coffin. I don't know what words passed between them. He finally turned away and, without looking at me, side-stepped toward the knots of visitors who had gathered in the doorway.

It was my turn. I stepped up to the coffin. Gram did not look as though she were sleeping, as people always said. She looked very dead, her square chin frozen in place, the gaunt cheeks slightly jaundiced under the powder, the wrinkles behind her glasses calcified. She seemed to have become a personification of her moniker: slight as a gram, less than an ounce. I felt I could reach into that coffin and pick her up with two fingertips, the way one might handle a dead sparrow on the windowsill. She had always made herself diminutive, had never wanted to be a bother. She had sat quietly in kitchen corners, or in the backseats of cars, always eager to listen, to listen to anything at all you might want to tell her.

The last time I had seen Gram alive, she had taken both my hands in hers in the foyer of her house. Somehow we stood alone together amidst the chaos of a family farewell, people gathering their hats and coats, impatiently waiting for each other or already stomping out the door. I remember the feel of those hands in mine, how strong they were, how dry. She gripped my hands so that I was forced to bend a little and look her straight in the eyes. Those eyes grew enormous behind her glasses, and pale, and in them I saw my own reflection. "I can't wait for you to be a part of this family," she said. She said it, I think now, in a fierce whisper, and the words hung in that foyer, with its beveled glass and umbrella stand, the coatrack behind her giving off a smell of body heat and Northern winters, even in the fall.

She was one of those legion of women who have locked me into the orbit of their families with a steady glance, a knowing look, a secretive handshake under the kitchen table. Grandmothers cling to me often this way, sensing either their grandsons' emotional infirmities, or my own tendencies toward flight. The grandmothers, one step removed from the core of the family, recognize in me what no one else dares. They put their thin arms around my waist like ropes, as if to tether me to the family, to keep me in one place. They cup their hand to my cheek and gaze into my eyes as if I were a precious newborn. It is precisely these women I hesitate to leave, when I contemplate leaving men—even more so, sometimes, then the man himself.

"Me, too," I squeezed back, "maybe soon." Then someone honked a horn, or came angling through the doorway, and I turned before she could see me cry. Because even as I squeezed her hand in reassurance, I knew Keith would never be my husband; even the word "husband," when I said it aloud, came husky from my throat; it buzzed in my mouth and did strange things to my lips and my tongue. What is this love that feels more keen for the knowledge of its own demise? It seems to me, now, it's the only kind of love I've known, the only kind I trust.

I bent nearer to the open coffin, expecting the odor of formaldehyde or flowers, but all I could smell was her dress—that blue polyester imbued with the scent of her closet: a dry smell, full of wood and camphor and long plastic bags keeping things new. I thought of her life, so cramped it seemed just then: those small rooms on the second floor, the childhood spent with cousins, a husband who died young. Perhaps I touched that waxy hand, briefly, and then snatched my own hand away. I can't honestly say.

Perhaps I leaned close to her ear, that ear always cocked for a kind word, for a familiar footstep to return home, and I murmured whatever I knew. I gave assurances. I think I said I loved her, words I'd rarely spoken even to my own grandmothers, whose deaths were imminent, whose funerals, it turned out, I would not attend. But to Gram, I promised whatever I could.

Afterward we stood about the room, milling in small groups as if at a cocktail party. People—neighbors and cousins—came in the front door, walked up to the coffin, paused, then walked away and began talking to us about the weather, Keith's plans for the future, Amy's acting gigs, small-town politics. And Gram sat in the corner, in her good dress, just listening, her head tilted a little to the left on its satin pillow, her hair curled in a perfect gray oval around her face. I kept glancing over at her, wondering what she would make of such a gathering. She would have been pleased, I think, at the lack of fuss, at the flow of normal conversation circling around her well-groomed self. She would have been quite happy to be here among us, inconspicuous, not yet alone.

The turnout in the church was respectable enough, the pews half full, a reverent hush in the room. The coffin, now closed on the altar, sat with Gram's body neatly inside it, the limbs folded and tucked. A minister who had never met Gram presided over the service, leading us in a recitation of Psalm 23: "The Lord is my shepherd, I shall not want...." I could sense Keith beside me in the pew; he remained still, but I could feel his anger rising, palpable as heat. I could see his profile, his jaw rigid, his eyes blinking rapidly behind his glasses. Gram was a woman, Keith would emphasize later in his eulogy, who had felt excluded from church and God, who always felt the outsider, standing on tiptoe to gaze through the streaked windows.

I watched Keith uncrimp himself from the pew and make his way to the dais. I watched that beloved forehead furrow in grief and speak of the woman I already missed so keenly. And I knew, even then, that I, too, was an outsider, a woman who would never quite fit into this family. As I engaged in this funeral and all its accompanying maneuvers—the plane tickets, the solemn conversations with his father, the shared bedroom with the full-length mirrors, the standing shoulder-to-shoulder at the viewing, the sitting shoulder-to-shoulder in the church—I relished the role of wife, even going so far as to straighten the knot in Keith's tie. But I remained aware of a separate, prophetic self: one who stood aside, made clucking noises in her throat, and whispered that I was an impostor.

Perhaps I had always seen my own fears magnified in Gram's eyes, and that's why I felt so bereft now at her absence, my compadre in silent alarm. I could project myself years into the future, alone on a bed, with no son, no grandson, to watch for my last breath. I'd been reading Alfred Kazin's memoir *A Walker in the City* and was haunted by these lines: "The most terrible word was *aleyn*, alone. I always had the same picture of a man desolately walking down a dark street, newspapers and cigarette butts contemptuously flying in his face as he tasted in the dusty grit the full measure of his strangeness." Already I could see myself as that stranger, untethered from the safe moorage of family. So as I watched Keith stand uncertainly behind the podium, speaking for Gram, I tried to catch his eye; I nodded my head vigorously to let him know I was there. But the light was dim, the chapel large, and I might have blended in my brown dress into the dusty wood of the pews.

Keith helped carry Gram's coffin to the graveside. She had been so tiny, so frail, I was surprised to see how hard the men had to work, their shoulders straining at the load, their faces flushing from the effort. When they reached the grave, someone stumbled and the coffin teetered a bit before it hit the ground. Everyone jumped forward, hands outstretched, as if to catch her, but the coffin rocked and settled on its own. As we stood waiting for the burial, Terry let his gaze rest on the tombstone. He let out a stifled cry, something between a groan and an "Oh, no," and I turned to follow his gaze. They had gotten Gram's name wrong, etched the word "Elizabeht" into the granite.

That's when I began to cry. I thought of Gram carrying her misspelled self into eternity, standing on tiptoe outside the gates of paradise. "Just looking," she might say to whoever asked, and they would leave her there, mispronounced and alone.

I'm wearing Gram's kimono this morning, the first time this season. Just now it seems meant for a woman much smaller than I am, a woman with more delicate bones, finer skin, a purer heart. It falls open at the knees, bunches a little at my breasts. The finches, when they swoop to rest on the porch rails, seem to eye the red vines with interest, sidestepping their way toward me. I see now the vines are really loose clusters of lotus blossoms floating across a pond, each one connected to the other by slender filaments. These flowers don't quite bloom; they seem to hesitate, as if waiting for each other before continuing to grow.

As I sit here in company with the finches, I think of Gram and the family I came so close to joining. Since then, there have been several clans like hers, families that call me to join them, to become wife, mother, daughter-in-law. I've just left another one behind, a grandmother who squeezed my hand under the dining room table and hoarsely whispered, "You're such a blessing to this family." But for reasons I can't articulate, I've not yet been able to stay; I seem inept at wearing the guises other women don with apparent ease. Family, right now, seems a country quite far from me, one that requires new sets of clothing styled for foreign climes.

Each year the robe gets dingier, the sleeves more yellowed, the hem frayed, the red blossoms a paler shade of red. But still, I wrap it tightly around me, tie the belt in a little square knot, and mull on the word "kimono" a name that sounds so right for this raiment: so full and rich, a word that makes the mouth pucker as if for a kiss. Perhaps, like Keith, I believe in the power of language to clarify. If we use the right words, then the world might suddenly align itself, become knowable and good. Here's a word I recently learned: "decouple," which means to separate; it's meant for electricians, this verb to describe the simple act of disattachment. But of course I want to appropriate the word for my own uses, to verbalize the way it feels to move from being a couple and back to living as a single woman. But it still does not carry the meaning I want, the sense of detaching from an entire family, to disengage oneself from that magnetic circle. "Defamily"? No, the word already exists: it is "defamiliarize." I seize this word to describe how it feels to slip out of a family—to become a stranger, out of kilter, almost alien.

I haven't spoken with Keith in several years. I know he's married now, with two children, but of his life and his family I have hardly an inkling. Yet every time I put on Gram's robe, there is a moment when I think of us going into that darkened bedroom after the funeral, leaving the rest of the family to their troubles. We open the door and see the kimono, bright as ever, winking in the recesses of her closet. Keith slips the robe gently from its hanger—it makes barely a sound—and hands it to me without a word. He knows it's the only thing I want, the only gift I need to take away.

Season of the Body

How good it's been to slide back
the heart's hood awhile, how fortunate
there's a heart and a covering for it,
and that whatever is still warm
has a chance.

—Stephen Dunn

I.

OCTOBER 1, THE FIRST DAY OF HUNTING SEASON in Wyoming, and I wear a fluorescent orange cap wherever I go, smug in the knowledge that my human heart this month makes me more sacred than a deer's running flanks. The deer graze close to the road, jerk their heads up to stare and freeze for the few moments it would take, if I had a gun, to set them clearly in my sights. Only then do they run, noiselessly sailing over sage and alfalfa, their white tails giving them away. A pickup full of shotguns passes. The orange cap bobs on my head, says *I am human, I am human,* and it's a relief, somehow, to have it all so clear today, the demarcations so sharp: who is edible and who is not.

But the next day I'll forget my orange cap. I'll stand at the edge of the field, my animal heart beating and beating. For some reason I'm wearing wild turkey feathers in my breast pocket and so I rustle when I move, a hunted thing. I'm wearing pants the color of sagebrush, a shirt the brown of new leather. I know I'm asking for it. I feel myself in their sights, appraised for the tone of my skin, the structure of my bones.

I'll make it out alive. We'll eat roast pheasant for dinner. The meat, when I tear it with my teeth, tastes faintly of sage, tastes of what they fed on, these iridescent birds in the underbrush. I nibble the meat from the bone, grind it between my molars, swallow. I keep eating and eating, can't stop, can't put a halt to my hunger, not so much for the meat but for the afterthought of sage, for what seasons the meat as it grows. I sit back at the table, my fingernails bright with grease, and wonder what I'll taste like when they finally get me. Will I have a bouquet of chocolate, the faintest waft of cinnamon? The sour-sweet tang of French bread and butter? I once saw twelve antelope strung up in my landlord's garage. He took a slice from each of them, grilled the meat so we could taste each one, find the bad ones in the batch, the ones that stank of fear.

Think of roasted garlic, Kalamata olives, Asiago cheese. Think of green chilies, poblanos, the snap of red pepper. Think of how your pores open during sex. Think of yourself drunk on good champagne, or the glass of Chardonnay like a bell on your tongue. Think of these odors wafting through you as an aftertaste, the taste that comes after you're gone.

II.

Once, in the summer of 1982, we shot a deer by the banks of the Big River. We shot him because he refused to move, refused to make it easy on all of us and migrate downriver to another garden, one with more roses than ours, or perhaps a garden with the sweet flowers of marijuana to make him mellow, let him roll around in the grass and forget about jumping fences. This was California after all, Mendocino county, and the gardens there were potent, hidden, cash crops with buds pungent as sex, sticky and warm. But the deer, a puritan, liked our roses better and Seth tracked him upstream, found the hole in the fence, fixed it, but still the deer wiggled in and ate the buds, nibbled the blossoms off the newborn squash. If this kept up, we'd have no food, no beauty that year.

So Seth borrowed a gun, who knows what kind, and tracked the deer again, saw him against the fence, too complacent to run, sated with the sugar of roses. His hunger made us angry, though it was common hunger, instinctual. Seth shot him clean through the chest. He told me how the deer buckled, fell to its knees as if in a last-ditch effort at apology.

Seth ate the heart that night. Maybe it was the liver, but I prefer to remember it as the heart, slices of it sautéed in butter and garlic, a bit of thyme. He ate it as a kind of restitution. He'd read that when Native American hunters killed a bear, they ate the heart right out of its chest, still beating. It went well with a bit of French bread, a salad of wild greens. At night I heard rustling in the garden and expected to see Seth on all fours among the roses, nibbling the folded petals, stepping delicately among the thorns.

But more often than not it was the raccoons, their eyes blinking at the open window, their human hands guilty on the compost.

III.

If you go to an acupuncturist complaining of heart trouble, he might turn your forearm pale-side up, trace the pericardial meridian with his fingertips. He'll start at your wrist and glide his finger across the dip of your elbow, the declination of a shoulder. "The pericardium," he tells you, "is the organ from which the feeling of happiness comes." He knows that what protects the heart brings the most pleasure. Not the heart itself, which is too meaty, too practical for love, beating and beating inside the sac. Cells of heart muscle cultured in a dish will beat on their own, thoughtlessly, ferocious, even with no body to sustain.

Close your eyes and your body has no bounds. Or it is all sheath, all skin, holding what balks at being contained. Trace the meridian all the way to the breastbone, return the way that you came: a brush of the shoulder, a swoon of the elbow, a question mark on the wrist. Wait for the needle, patiently, the way you might wait for a kiss.

Or pretend you're in another kind of doctor's office, one where they enter the body and take away a vial of blood. Feel your arm in the same position: open, flat against the steel table, so pale it's gone luminous. Blood runs close to the surface here, that's why it hurts so much and feels so good when they hand you the clean cotton ball and you press it to the wound and bend.

IV.

Admit it. What we want is to get at the heart: not the metaphorical heart, not the heart that is symmetrical and good-natured and red.

We want to lay a finger on the unthinking muscle, the beating core of the body. Writing for *The New York Times Magazine*, Charles Siebert describes holding a transplanted heart in his hand. "I was expecting to feel a kind of gelatinous warble," he writes, "but got instead these hot, firm, repeated blows against my palm, the force resonating up my arm. I can feel them still." It's a language that exists before the tongue; feel your own tongue rising to drink it.

After Rhea gave birth to Sean, she ate a bit of the placenta. The meat of it looked like heart muscle to me, glossy, bright. I touched it in the special ceramic bowl; it felt like the living flesh of someone's abdomen. Rhea sautéed it in butter and onions. I watched her. She took tiny bites, chewing carefully. *This is my body,* I thought I heard her say. *Eat of it and be healed.*

V.

When they gutted their first chicken, Rhea told me, she saw the eggs, all the eggs the chicken would lay in her life, spiraled inside a sac: the largest egg at the lip, then decreasing in size until they clustered as a mass of microbes in the core. The shells, she said, were opalescent as pearls. All of them intact and edible, for someone with fingers and lips delicate enough to touch them without breaking.

She tells me this, describes the egg spiral with her hands, while we're camped in Kodachrome Basin in southern Utah. In the cooler we have "farm fresh" eggs bought from a Mormon family in Cannon-ville, brown and enormous, waiting to be soft-boiled in the morning, their shells rough like sandpaper against my fingertips. We bought them from two boys playing in their yard. We stopped at Bryce Valley Supply where the lights were off and the salsa jars sat dusty on the shelf. We thought *soft-boiled eggs with salsa and toast* in the morning, and already the meal existed, already we longed for the yolk of eggs melting on the bread, wanted the night to be done with so we could eat.

The campground has been taken over by a convocation of teen-aged girls. They are lovely and exasperating, whinnying to each other on the way to and from the bathroom. They stand a long time disapproving of themselves in the bathroom mirrors, their eyes narrow, their thin hands fluttering about their faces, touching one invisible blemish and then another. Their thighs are smooth and brown and hairless—no scars, no bites, no veins. They wait in line for the shower; they twirl bits of hair around their index fingers. They spread their makeup kits along the narrow counter; some have many compartments holding creams, lotions, and pots of dusty pigment.

I think of their eggs, inside them already, in a spiral, weightless as bubbles.

The girls have chaperones. They stand outside the bathroom, forever waiting for the girls to be done, but they will never be done, they will continue their ablutions forever in the damp, fogged mirrors. Rhea and I have no chaperone except for "Big Stony," a mammoth, penis-shaped rock above campsite #17. The girls, I think, take no notice of it, their vision narrowed down to the path between campsite and bathroom, but we joke about the rock's anatomical correctness: the rounded arrowhead of the tip, the two testicles anchoring the phallus to the mesa. When night falls the penis looms above us, pointing toward the stars. It demands sacrifice and worship, the silhouette like a God of Sensual Longing, a God who wants and wants without surcease.

That night I dream of something that wakes me crying "No!" I look outside the tent, and Big Stony towers in the moonlight, unmoved, unchanged. The girls do not sleep but spiral through the campground in their chaperones' cars, desperate for a mirror.

In the morning I wake and soft-boil the eggs, time them for exactly three minutes, while the chukars come out of hiding. They are partridges from Asia, with crowned heads, a low coo, brought to this desert for decoration. They strut in the damp morning dirt, clucking for bits of lettuce, the discarded rinds of fruit.

When the eggs are done I crack the shells and scoop out their soft hearts with a spoon.

VI.

My hunger knows no bounds. Yours, too, my dear, I see it beating in your gums. My what big teeth you have, bigger than a newborn's heart, which is only one inch wide, weighs under an ounce. How easy it would be to swallow such a heart if you could get to it.

The infant I care for, Emma, knows the world through her mouth, holds my lips with her fingers, touches my dangerous teeth. I touch her heart with my fingertip when she sleeps, to make sure she's still alive. When she wakes, she pries open my mouth, looks fearlessly into the abyss of my hunger, tries to put her whole head into that yawning expanse. *I could eat you up,* I growl to her, and she laughs.

VII.

When I was a small child of seven or eight I watched my mother make chopped liver. She made it every year for Hanukkah, and I remember her gutting the chicken with her bare hands. I saw her at the kitchen counter, saw her right hand hold down the carcass, her left hand enter that dark cavern. I thought how convenient for the entrails to emerge so nicely packaged and bound with string. At that age I had no clear idea of the arrangement of my own viscera (I still don't—looking at a diagram in the *Encyclopedia Britannica* I'm shocked to discover my liver so enormous, bigger than my heart and so near it, way up in the top strata of my rib cage). This package both humbled and horrified me. She pulled out the neck, the gizzards, the heart. She pulled out the cubes of liver, added extra ones from a plastic tub in the fridge, fried them in chicken fat with onions, chopped them with a cleaver and mixed them with boiled eggs, mayonnaise, a little salt, a little pepper. She set the bowl out on the counter next to a platter of thickly sliced *challah*, a bread the color of yolk.

We ate it quickly, scooping up big gobs of chopped liver with torn hunks of bread, mumbling our pleasure through full mouths. Yet whenever any of us felt rejected, underappreciated, we raised our voices and exclaimed: *"So what am I, chopped liver?"* as if chopped liver were something negligible. I heard my grandfather shout it to my grandmother in their bedroom in Brooklyn. I heard my father laugh it to my mother in the kitchen in Los Angeles. I repeated it on my way to school, my feet kicking the leaves on the sidewalk. *What am I, chopped liver? What am I?* The mere mention of chopped liver set my mouth watering, and then, in this transfiguring chant, I *became* the dish, a conflation that made me dizzy with words, with hunger, my body a sudden and accidental source of satiation.

VIII.

It's not just the animal body I want, the mathematics of sex, the coupling: I want another heart, an extra one, a contrabassoon to echo my everyday pulse. It's not my imagination. I hear it there, beating inside me. My bones pop and creak in their sockets.

IX.

Hunger does not belong to the belly. Even those with stomachs removed still feel hunger loose within their bodies, pangs in the abdomen, the tongue. Scientists, despite prodding the various centers of the brain, do not know where hunger lives, have yet to discover precisely hunger's location. It is not a finger on the inner lining of the heart. It is not a tooth grating on the esophagus.

But they know this hunger starts in utero. In the womb, we drink what our mother's bodies create. We drink the fluid in which we float, regulating the amnion in perfect equilibrium. In utero, breathing, drinking, eating: all the same, an orgy of consumption. And even as a fetus we know the bitter from the sweet, and we choose the one with sugar in it. Sometimes the amniotic fluid goes bitter, the fetus will refuse to drink, and the solution, unregulated, swells in the uterus, creating a fatal condition. Both mother and child will die.

So do not fault me for my sweet tooth; it's what we use to survive. Do not complain if you find me among the rosebushes, nibbling the amber petals. Do not fault me for my thirst, my hunger, my desire to absorb every delectable thing. *This is my body,* a voice nudges you in the dark. *Drink of it and be healed.*

X.

And when you finally eat me, when your hunger can no longer be contained, start with my arm. Mouth the little curves that lead to the pericardium. Turn my wrist to trace the subcutaneous secrets of my heart. Be a phlebotomist: extract this double evidence of life and desire. Find the Auricle, Ventricle, Vein. The Arch of Aorta, Superior Vena Cava, beating behind their glossy shield. Probe for the fluid of the womb, sip it, I swear it will be sweet.

XI.

Yes, love, here are my bones. Gnaw them until they gleam.

EPILOGUE

"... what I would like to capture aren't thoughts but the scent of my happiness..."

—Jacques Henri Latrique

LATELY I'VE TAKEN TO WRITING BACKWARD in my notebook: not the sentences, themselves, but the pages—back to front—as if I mean to write a Jewish prayer book, a *Midrash* to answer my own sacred questions. I remember, in my childhood, sitting in the synagogue on Friday evenings, the weight of such a book on my lap, the black covers (so thick, so impenetrable!) pointed in the wrong direction. I ran my fingertips along the gilded edges of the pages, riffling them a little to release their musty smell. The pages felt so different from ordinary books—thin as tissue, easily torn—and I must have known, even without my parents' admonitions, that such a book must be handled with care, with reverence.

But each time I opened the covers, moments before the religious doldrums set in, I felt more anticipation than awe. To begin where the ending should be, and move in reverse—it all felt so wrong, so foreign, so *arousing*. My brain—the part just behind my forehead— seemed to stretch a little in its cage, releasing some anodyne that made my ears tingle. I heard the entire congregation turn the pages in synch, and watched how their fingertips barely stroked the written words as they followed along with the cantor. With each turn of the page I thought *now* I might understand: what existed *back there*, in the recesses of the book? What kind of answer might be revealed in this slow, backward motion of prayer?

Perhaps I was so intrigued by the Jewish prayer books because, in my daily life, I read voraciously in the "normal" way, front-to- back, like someone addicted to stories. I checked out ten books at a time from the local library and read them in my small bedroom, oblivious to the sunny, suburban backyard outside my window. The gap between language and sense dissolved, and I simply *under- stood*, with little thought or effort. If the story were particularly good, I found myself slowing down near the finale, my thumb and fore- finger resting a long while on the tip of the penultimate page before gradually, reluctantly, turning. Out the corner of my eye I saw the white space at the bottom of the last page, an abyss that signaled the end. It was, perhaps, my first experience of the bittersweet quality of endings, that tug between loss and the sweet desire such loss engenders.

When I finally closed the back cover I held my palm flat against its surface a while, as if divining some vibration, some message still emanating from within the pages. Sometimes, after a decent interval had passed, I turned the book over and opened it again to page one. I perused the first paragraph, gratified to know the beginning still existed—intact, but transformed by time and the knowledge of what would come.

While I read I believed, without knowing it, in the certitude of narrative: that all beginnings inevitably lead to some kind of conclusion. I believed a story began at some predetermined point in time and moved steadily forward toward its inborn resolution. These two parts did not change—the beginning remained the beginning, the conclusion remained the end—no matter how often I read the stories, or how long I stayed away. I found a stunning comfort in this symmetry, this permanence. And I translated the patterns of literature into my own life, narrating my experiences even as they occurred: I pinpointed beginnings, traced the arc of narrative, strove for neat resolutions, threads tied up, and lessons learned for good.

But now, as I write backward in my notebook, I've come to think such an enterprise is hardwired for failure; after all, do we ever live our lives as determinedly *forward* as our narratives suggest? Don't we all find ourselves doubling back, playing out the same plots again and again, each time with their strangely unsatisfying conclusions? These endings never stay put, but keep changing into beginnings; eventually we're left reeling in a perpetual present, one that begs off the question of where the past ends and the future begins.

I'm writing backward in my notebook in Oaxaca, Mexico, on a rooftop terrace with my godson Sean. We're writing together as the morning lightens around us. We're in a high valley surrounded by peaks just now growing visible in the haze. Closer in, I focus on pots of gardenias and bougainvillea dotting the roof's ledge. We are strangers here, my godson and I; we sit under a Mexican sky, overlaid with wisps of Mexican clouds, and the trees are Mexican:

Acacias and Eucalyptus. The tile roofs are Mexican, and the adobe walls, and the bulldog who stands sentinel on the rooftop next door. The water man pushes his laden cart through the streets, his voice a song: *Agua, Agua,* two bass notes that reverberate in the cobblestone alleys. Next door, a woman fries tortillas on a blackened griddle; she fills them with soft cheese and hot peppers. There are roosters crowing and dogs barking, a broom sweeping over wet stones in the courtyard.

Here, in Oaxaca, I'm introduced everywhere as Sean's *madrina,* and people smile at me in approval, nodding their heads, turning from me to him as if they see a thin rope linking godmother to godson. In Oaxaca, the godmother becomes a second mother, sharing the child and all its joys and burdens. In Judaism, the godmother carries the infant to the altar for the circumcision; it is she who presents the child into a covenant with God. I wish I could claim such responsibility: for me, godmother has always been an honorary title; I've done nothing, really, to deserve it but bear witness to Sean's birth, to hold him long into the night when he cried as a baby. But here, in this country, the word has taken on weight, as if Sean and I are connected not with a physical umbilicus, but by a cord made of some finer substance, one that links us at the heart.

I look up and glance sidelong at Sean. He's bent to his notebook, gripping his pen in his hands the way he did when he was just a child. His blond bangs—thick and gold, like his mother's—fall over his eyes; he has one long ponytail slithering down his back. He's almost seventeen, and enormous, towering above both me and his mother, but most often he slouches, keeping his hands buried deep in the pockets of his baggy shorts. He's an excellent traveler, talking in fluent Spanish to the boys his age we meet on the street. I don't know what he says to them, but their faces light up when they speak together; they lean heads close to examine a map, or merely stand nodding together in that smug surety teen-agers have, so pleased at their language, their brief communiqués.

Sean looks up from his notebook and off into the distance, tapping his pen on the glass rim of the table. Though he's not looking at me, I can still see in his face the two-year-old I adored: the fat cheeks, the raised eyebrows, the broad smile. It will never disappear, that beloved face; it will never go away, even as he ages into an old man. As I gaze at him, I think about the other children I've loved: children like Hannah and Sarah, or those babies I held on the Infant Ward. I imagine the faces of my own children: what would I have seen if I looked in their eyes? Would they have narrated a story that goes back to my great-grandmother Bluma, standing with folded arms in the kitchen garden of her house in Romania? Would I have seen my own face as an infant, the child mirroring back to me my own beginnings? I don't know, but for a brief moment I think I understand what sustains the love between mothers and sons, fathers and daughters: it's the imprint of those faces on our memories, the child always a child, no matter how much he grows.

I look back down to my notebook, turn another page, keep writing in this backward-facing script. I think about those narratives I loved so much as a child, with their good faith in an orderly progression, their clear beginnings and their emphatic "The End." To me, these days, story is more about *continuance,* the ways we keep coming back, the ways we keep going on. As I write, I feel my past selves loitering inside me: a girl listening to the ringing telephone at her hospital bedside; a young woman sitting cross-legged in meditation for days at a time; a massage therapist cupping her hands on the holy bone. These younger selves, and many others, conspire to make me what I am at this moment: a forty-one-year-old woman, single and childless, writing with her godson in the light of a Oaxacan morning. Her body feels composed, corrected, as if reeled in from some wayward path. She hears the faint ring of a bell at the front gate of the posada, and the shuffle of feet bringing *chocolate caliente* and *pan dulce* to the breakfast table. In a little while she'll close her notebook and go down into the streets alone. She'll wander into the neighborhood church—with its peeling frescos, its splintered doorframe—and watch three matrons kneel at the altar to sing their rosaries to Mary, the mother of all their beliefs.

I won't know the language; for that I'll need Sean as a guide. But I'm learning there are limits to what can be told, even in languages we think we know so well. I'll understand enough to stand quietly in the background, hands folded at my belly, my body resonant with prayer.

The Author

Brenda Miller is an Assistant Professor of English at Western Washington University. She has received two Pushcart Prizes for her work in creative nonfiction, and her essays have been published in periodicals such as *The Sun, Utne Reader, Prairie Schooner, The Georgia Review,* and *Seneca Review.* Her work has been anthologized in *The Beacon Best of 1999: Creative Writing by Women* 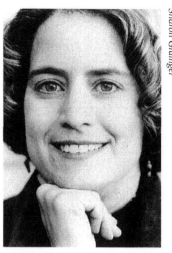 *and Men of All Colors; Storming Heaven's Gate: An Anthology of Spiritual Writings by Women;* and *In Brief: Short Takes on the Personal.* She is Editor-in-Chief of *The Bellingham Review.*